Lucien G Prince, MD, MBA,MS-CVRT, CLVT

Inside The Eye
DISEASE

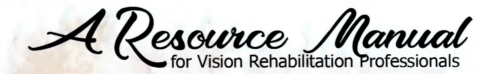

A Resource Manual for Vision Rehabilitation Professionals

By: Lucien G. Prince, MD, MBA-Healthcare Mgt, MS-CVRT, CLVT

DEDICATION: To all Clients with blindness or visual impairments who inspired me to get back to the field.

To order additional copies of this book, contact:
Xlibris
1-888-795-4274
www.Xlibris.com
Orders@Xlibris.com

ISBN: Softcover   978-1-7960-8397-2
        Hardcover   978-1-7960-8398-9
        EBook   978-1-7960-8396-5

Library of Congress Control Number: 2020901068

Print information available on the last page.

Rev. date: 01/21/2020

Preface

The majority of Vision Rehabilitation Professionals who teach clients how to use their remaining field of view is constantly asked to recommend the right book to explain eye diseases. Although, there are several great textbooks on the visual field available, none seems to meet the standard that rehabilitation professionals require to satisfy their clients' needs. This book is therefore the prescription that encompasses the major topics of eye disease in relation to low vision, orientation, mobility and vision therapy. This book answers all the questions about the anatomy, physiology, pathophysiology, pathology, treatment, prevention and vision rehabilitation therapy of any abnormality of the eye. This book can serve as a companion text for not only for vision rehabilitation professionals but also medical students and family members of patients. The audience includes certified optometrists and ophthalmologists; pediatric and occupational MDs and RNs; allied health personnel in ophthalmology and optometry and pharmacists. It may also be of interest to those involved in a wide range of occupations in industry, government, military and civil aviation and maritime functions. It aims to help fulfill the thirst for knowledge about functional visual impairment and blindness.

I would like to express my gratitude to my CFO Jeanine Johnson and the numerous contributors that made this text possible:
- Lachelle E. Smith, M.S., CVRT (Director of the Vision Rehabilitation Therapist Program Salus University)
- Audrey Smith, PHD (Dean, College of Education and Rehabilitation, Salus University, Professor, Blindness and Low Vision)
- Krystell D. Prince, MSc. (Clinical Data Analyst)
- Eric G. Austin (Media/Marketing)
- Jerline Aristide(Intern)
- Vision Rehabilitation Staff at EBRC (Eastern Blind Rehab Center, West Haven, CT VA Facility)
- VISIONS Rehab Staff and Management (New York, NY)

Foreword

Although blindness has existed since the beginning of recorded history, it became a major societal concern after World War II, when the hospitals were filed with visually impaired veterans. The strong, brave men and women, who had so valiantly fought for world peace and human rights, were now perceived as weak and helpless. It was at that time the rehabilitation professionals began to analyze the issues of living without sight. As of today, the majority of the population still see individuals with visual impairment as someone who has lost psychological security, basic skills, communication skills (reading, writing), and appreciation of all that is beautiful. They are also believed to have lost control over their financial occupational status and personality. However, while many perceived people who are visually impaired or blind as helpless, resentful, bitter and unhappy, some advocate that blindness itself does not create emotional disturbance. Instead, it is societal prejudices that cause emotional distress; it is the misconceptions about the loss of vision or the need for adaptive skills that causes the anxiety (Cutsforth 1951: Jernigan, 1969).

Although, there is a lot of progress in the evolution of attitudes and stereotypes towards disability and visual impairment in the U.S population, the ancient misconceptions still exist. Individuals who are blind or visually impaired are still being regarded in some part of the society as a different class of people with definite stereotyped characteristics. The loss of vision is still looked upon as punishment by many; for example, parents may feel guilty that their child visually impaired. Also, very often the parents of blind children get the impression from physicians and nurses that the child will be hopeless and helpless. This is a great dis-service because, without a good understanding of the child's capabilities, the child will not succeed in life.

Being the Chief Medical Officer for a Medical and Paramedical Exam Company for over 14 years, I received a full range of cases of individuals with multiple disabilities including blindness/ visual impairment. These people had no idea about the severity of their eye's conditions and thought they were going to regain their sight. They are helpless if their families do not have the financial resources to send them to a low vision or blind rehab facility. To quote one of them: "I *don't want to go to restaurants with my husband anymore, because I don't want to embarrass him with his friends*". There is a disbelief and recognition and emotions over there. Very often, nurses working in hospitals or nursing homes tend to collect medical information needed from the visually impaired or blind client's companion instead of asking the client directly. In addition, a person may be called "blind" when he/she lacks common sense and "stolen blind" when someone foolishly allows himself/herself to be cheated. Other terms such as blind alley, blind fury, intellectually blind or morally blind, all have negative connotations affect the population with which I'm working. This presents a real challenge in the rehabilitation process. Bad pirates still wear eye patches in storybooks or movies, while physical beauty is constantly advertised over the media. The strangest assumption commonly held is that as soon as a person becomes blind or visually impaired, he/she immediately takes on all the stereotypical characteristics. To quote Helen Keller:" *not blindness, but the attitude of the seeing to the blind is the hardest burden* to bear". Generally, the society is geared to accommodate the majority and thus the needs of these minorities are often forgotten. The society reinforce dependency of individuals diagnosed with blindness or vision loss; they assist them with service systems that make it unnecessary to compete for their survival needs. The fact is, of course that some people with vision loss can survive in our competitive society on their own, but many cannot without support.

As a Vision Rehab Specialist, it will be important that we not only educate the general public about blindness and disability, but also the blind person's family, friends and associates. In addition, the individual who is blind or visually impaired will have to learn through training how to effectively manage negative encounters. While assisting clients in their adaptation to visual impairment, we must view ourselves as positive role models and **know that the client is a person first.** In other words, we must play a positive role by changing the attitudes of both sighted and visually impaired or blind clients. It will be important to encourage individual with vision loss to be taught together with the sighted whenever possible.

All these memories along with some Alumni from Salus University motivate me to come back to the vision field and finish what being already started. The personal satisfaction you obtain from assisting individuals who are visually impaired, or blind is an indescribable fulfillment.

Being a practicing Low Vision Rehab Specialist, I have a better understanding of feelings, attitudes and recognize the impact that any negative feeling might have on individuals who are blind or visually impaired. I understand that attitudes of significant others (i.e. family and friends) have the most significant impact on a client's self-concept; families with positive attitudes most likely will help the individual who is blind or visually impaired maintain a positive outlook. To best understand the adjustment to vision loss, it is necessary first to be aware of the relationship between self-esteem and adjustment and to the concept of acceptance of loss. A good understanding of this book will give the eye care professionals the skills needed to assess clients diagnosed with visual impairment and blindness; the age at which vision loss occurred, the degree of vision loss and the coping strategies to use.

Contents

Chapter 1:
Understanding the Anatomy and Physiology of the eye

To understand the visual process, it is important to master the major parts of the eye, where the visual information is collected and transmitted. A thorough foundation on ocular anatomy will enable you to better understand diseases of the eye as well as the functional and educational implications of those anomalies and conditions.

Let's start with the anterior part (front) of the eye and way towards the back or posterior part. Images of different parts of the eye are provided to help with your learning.

The eye is a spherical organ. (Approximately one inch in diameter). It is suspended in a cone-shaped, bony structure called the **"orbit".** The bony orbits provide a safe shelter for the eyes. The eye detects energy (as photon) and transmits information about intensity, color and shape to the brain.

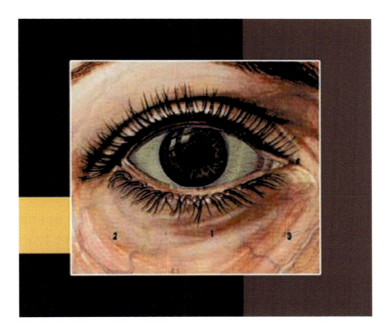

LIDS

The lids are a thin layer of epithelial tissue, which serves to protect the eye. The upper and lower lids are the thinnest layers of tissue in the body (see photo under conjunctiva section).

Functions:
- **Protects** eye from foreign bodies, dust
- Blinks as a **reflex**
- **Nourishes** cornea via its blood vessels
- Helps to **spread** tears
- **Limits** light entering the eye

LASHES
The lashes are hairs that insert into the margin (edge) or the upper and lower lids. The function is to protect the eye by catching dust and organisms and preventing them from entering the eye (see photo under conjunctiva section).

LACRIMAL SYSTEM
The **function** of the lacrimal system is to:
- Drain tears
- Produce tears via the lacrimal gland

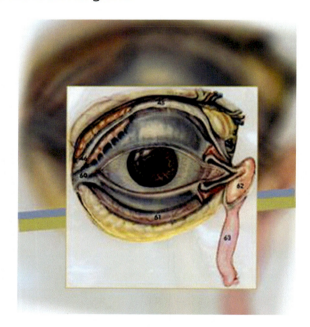

The lacrimal gland produces the tears, the lacrimal puncta (small opening in the inner lower and upper lids) collects the tears, the lacrimal sac further collect tears that drain into the nasolacrimal system. See the image above (62 is the lacrimal sac, 63 and 61 the lacrimal drainage systemal sac further collect tears that drain into the nasolacrimal system.

CONJUNCTIVA

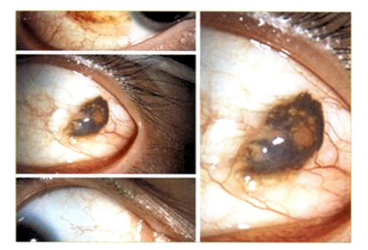

The conjunctiva is a thin mucoid translucent layer of cells that protect the eye.

- It lines the upper and lower lids, bulbar sclera (white part of the eye you can see) and ends at the cornea (the window to the eye).
- It contains blood vessels, which provide nutrition to the surface of the cornea. As far as functions, it protects the sclera from organisms and provide nutrition to the cornea.

Cornea:

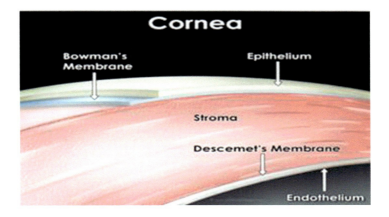

It is an extremely important structure of the eye because it is the key optical component responsible for refraction of light that enters the eye. It is an unusual tissue because it is clear and has no blood vessels. This explains why the cornea is susceptible to infection from bacterial, viral, fungal or allergic. The cornea is thicker at its periphery than at the center and is composed of six layers of tissue. The cornea is the protective "window" to the eye. It is highly refractive and bends light rays as they enter the eye. It has a convex surface that acts as a powerful lens. Like the crystal on a watch, it gives us a clear window to look through.

The cornea is **transparent** because of its:
- **Composition** – a regularly **arrangement** of collagen fibers (allowing individual light rays to pass between the fibers)
- **Avascular** nature - lack of blood vessels except for in the peripheral or limbal area
- **Hydration** level – a water content of 78% maintained by the endothelial cells

The cornea's **refractive** power is due to its **curvature**. It is curved like a convex lens. This is convex or plus (+) power that bends light rays together in a convergent way.

Note: a minus or concave lens bends light rays in a divergent way.

The cornea provides protection to the eye due to the characteristics of:

- Strength – one layer of the cornea is very strong and thus difficult to penetrate.
- Sensitivity – the cornea is highly innervated (lots of nerves). This high level of innervation means there are many pain receptors in the cornea. Pain alerts us to the danger of a foreign object, infections and so on.

The first structure in the visual pathway is the cornea. If the cornea is not transparent, less light will travel to the back of the eye (retina and optic nerve), and vision will be affected.

Sclera:

It is the thick fibrous outer layer, which serves as the protective coat of the eye. It contains 58-60% of water. The sclera also known as the white part of the eye provides durability and resistance to the wall of the eye. Place of attachment for extraocular muscles (EOM) and ciliary muscles. Beneath the sclera is the choroid layer, which helps to supply the retina with blood. It is dark, pigmented area that reduces reflection in the eye.

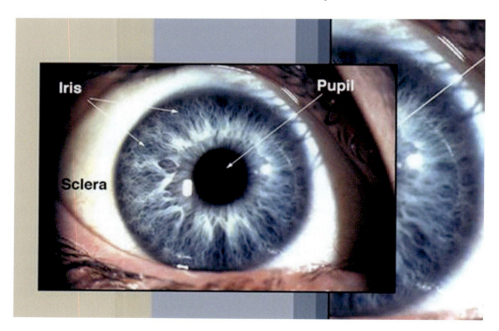

UVEAL TRACT (IRIS, CILIARY BODY, CHOROID) AND AQUEOUS

The uveal tract comprises the iris, ciliary body and choroid. These 3 related structures develop together prenatally. There is one common layer, which is continuous throughout the entire uveal tract (this makes it possible for infections, if untreated, to travel from the anterior to the posterior part of the eye).

Iris/Pupil:

Iris is considered as the colored ring like membrane suspended between the cornea and the lens. The amount of pigment determines the color of the eye (blue eyes have less pigment and brown eyes have more). In the center of the Iris is an opening called **the pupil,** through which light travels and is transmitted on the back of the eye. The Iris also contains a bundle of muscle fibers that control the size of the pupil, enabling it to constrict or dilate. For example, in bright light the pupil will constrict, affording protection from too much light or glare. In dim light the pupil will dilate, allowing as much light as possible to enter the eye

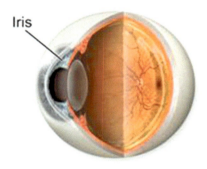

CILIARY BODY

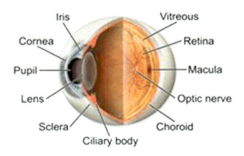

The Ciliary Body is in direct continuity with the Iris and is adherent to the "Sclera". Directly posterior to the Iris, the Ciliary Body is plump and thrown into numerous folds referred to as the "Ciliary Processes". This portion of the Ciliary Body is about 2.5 mm in length and is responsible for the major production of aqueous fluid. The posterior portion of the Ciliary body is flat and most of the Zonular Fibers of the lens originate from this structure of the Uveal Tract (Ciliary Body). Generally, the Ciliary Body is triangular, with its shortest side anterior. The anterior side of this triangle in its inner part enters the formation of the angle of the Anterior Chamber. From its middle portion the iris takes root. On the outer side of the triangle is the Ciliary Muscle, which lies against the sclera.

In this way, the Ciliary Body plays important roles in the health of the anterior segment of the eye:

- It is both a vascular and muscular structure with the dual function of producing aqueous fluid and through its muscles, controlling the shape of the lens. In other word, it controls accommodation by changing the shape of the crystalline lens. Usually when the ciliary body contracts, the Zonules relax. This allows the lens to thicken, increasing the eye's ability to focus up close. When looking at a distant object, the ciliary body relaxes, causing the Zonules to contract.
- It is instrumental in both nourishing the Cornea and Lens and controlling the Eye's focusing ability.

In children, the Ciliary Body muscle is extremely active, and the Lens is easily deformed, which accounts for its powerful range of accommodation, or focus abilities. The Ciliary muscle declines in power with age. This explains why people develops the condition known as "**presbyopia**" as they get older. This occurs as the ciliary body muscle and lens gradually lose elasticity, causing difficulty reading.

THE AQUEOUS

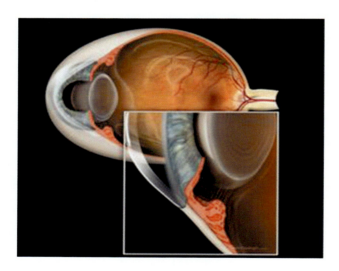

It is a water fluid that fills the front chambers of the eye in front of the lens but behind the cornea. The ciliary processes portion of the ciliary body produces aqueous daily. The aqueous chamber is the open space between the ciliary body and the endothelial layer of the cornea. The normal range of intraocular pressure (IOP) is related to the aqueous (production and outflow) in the eye.

Functions:
- **Nourishes** the cornea and lens
- Maintains **shape** of eye
- Maintains Intraocular **Pressure** (IOP)

Please be advised that:
1. The aqueous flows from the posterior to anterior portions of the aqueous chamber towards the angle via the trabecular meshwork to the canal of Schlemm into the vortex veins which is our venous drainage system
2. High IOP may be caused by too much aqueous being produced by the ciliary processes, not enough aqueous draining out of the angle (through the trabecular meshwork) or a combination of both production and outflow issues. Refer to the diagram above.
3. IOP is determined by the aqueous. High IOP MAY indicate glaucoma.

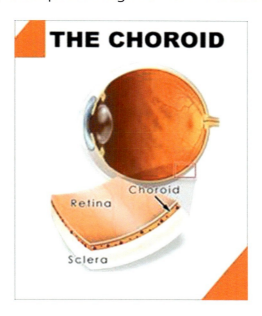

The choroid lies between the sclera and the retina. It is the **largest** part of the uveal tract (iris, ciliary body and choroid) and heavily **pigmented** (with melanin). It plays several roles:
- Serve as a **passageway** for nerves and vessels to the eye
- Provide a **dark screen** – attracting light to it.
- Provide a **smooth, regular surface** for photoreceptors
- Supply **blood/nourishment** to the outer 1/3 of retina
- Stabilize **ocular temperature**

THE LENS

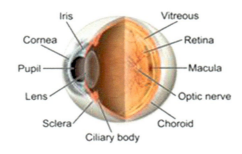

The Lens is a colorless and almost completely transparent flexible body which is suspended directly behind the iris by zonula fibers or suspensory ligament. It's convex and help bend light rays entered the eye through the cornea and passed through the pupil. The ciliary muscle controls the shape and focusing power of the lens. The lens also helps focus light rays on the retina. Composed of 65% water and 35% protein, the lens become larger and less elastic throughout life, which is the reason for **presbyopia** (a reduction in accommodative ability that occurs with age).

THE VITREOUS

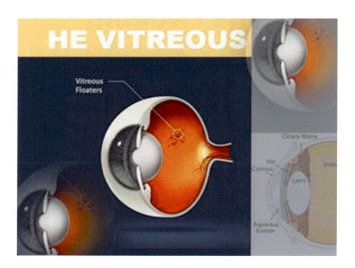

The **Vitreous:**
It's considered as a clear, avascular, jelly like substance which adheres to the back surface of the lens and to the back and sides of the eye. It enables the eye to maintain its shape and resilience. After light rays have been bent by the lens, they pass through the clear vitreous to the retina. It has minimal refractive power and is formed by the retina (prenatally, one time only)

Functions:
*   Maintains the shape of the eye
*   Transmits light
*   Provides a little nutrition to retina

The Retina and Optic Nerve Head

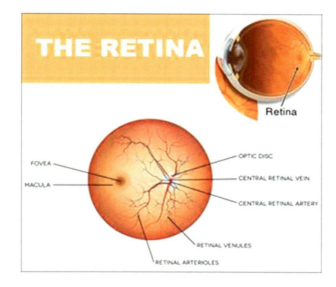

The Retina is the most internal coat of the eye. It is a thin delicate membrane with ten distinct layers of cells. It contains the sensory receptors for the transmissions of light. The retinal receptors are divided in two main populations: rods (function best in dim light) and cones (functions well under daylight conditions, color vision). The cones form a concentrated area in the retina known as the Fovea, which lies in the center of the macula. Whenever we look at an object, we must aim the eye so that the image of the object is focused on the Fovea. Smooth eye movement called pursuits and jump eye movements, called saccades are both designed to allow people to use the Fovea. So, the Retina serves to receive visual images and transmit information to the optical pathways of the brain through the optic nerve. In this way, light may pass through all layers of the retina to reach the photoreceptors where the visual process begins. Diseases like macular degeneration or diabetic retinopathy that affect the clarity of retina, or swelling that affects the shape of the retina, will have a profound effect on vision.

Reflection on functions of the 10 layers of the retina and how it enables a person to see colors:

The retina is a specialized neural tissue that lines the back of the eye. This tissue is responsible for capturing light and converting it to a chemical signal. There are ten layers of the retina and each serves a specific purpose in order to enable a person to see colors.

Retinal Pigmented Epithelium (RPE): is the last layer of the retina. It's a highly pigmented layer that absorbs excess light. The RPE serves as a nourishing and garbage –collecting layer for the photoreceptors. Its cells have very tight junctions between themselves, which prevent diffusion of substances between the choroidal circulation and the retina. This is the last layer of the retina and is attached to the structures behind the retina.

Photoreceptor: these are the rods and cones that receive light and undergo a chemical configuration change to detect light.

External Limiting Membrane: represents where the inner segments of the rods and cones are located. It's formed from adherens junctions between Muller cells and photoreceptor cell inner segments. It also forms a barrier between the sub retinal space, into which the inner and outer segments of the photoreceptors project to be in close association with the pigment epithelial layer behind the retina, and the neural retinal proper.

Outer Nuclear layer (ONL): these are the actual cell bodies of the rods and cones. It's about the same thickness in central peripheral retina. However, in peripheral rod, cell bodies outnumber the cone cell bodies which the reverse is true for central retina.

Outer Synaptic Layer or Outer Plexiform Layer (OPL): These are where the projections from the rods and cones synapse with the bipolar cells.

Inner Nuclear Layer (INL): contains the nuclei of the bipolar cells, horizontal and amacrine cells. The bipolar cells are responsible for relaying information from the photoreceptors to the ganglions.

Inner Synaptic Layer or Inner Plexiform Layer (IPL): is the area where the bipolar cells axons and the dendrites of the ganglion cells synapse. This area is where the two cells communicate. This is the area where the message concerning the visual image is transmitted to the brain along with the optic nerve.

Ganglion Cell Layer: contains nuclei of ganglion cells, the axons of which become the optic nerve fibers for messages and some amacrine cells. These ganglion cells are vital for transmitting the information from the photoreceptors to the brain. Damage to these cells will cause loss of vision.

Nerve Fiber Layer: is comprised of the axons of the ganglion's cells. Loss of nerve fibers can cause loss of vision, generally of the peripheral visions first before the central vision.

Internal Limiting Membrane: is the first structure light hits. It is the basement membrane for a cell called the Muller cell. The Muller cells serve as supporting structures for retinal ganglion cell complex. It is the inner surface of the retina forming a diffusion barrier between neural retina and vitreous humor.

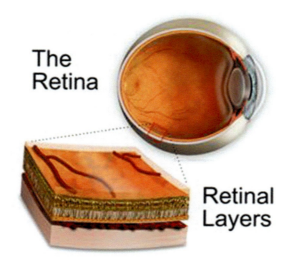

The Retina

Retinal Layers

How it enables a person to see colors:

In the retina, the photo sensitive cells like the rods and cones convert incident light energy into signals that are carried to the brain by the optic nerve. In the middle of the retina is a small dimple called the fovea or fovea centralis, which is the eye sharpest vision and the location of most color perception. In this way, a person can see colors when light is focused on fovea centralis or macula. This area has exclusively cones and they are smaller and more closely packed than elsewhere on the retina.

The Macula

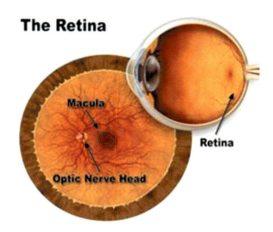

- Is the thinnest part of the retina
- The fovea, the center of the macula, provides the 20/20 acuity
- Is not fully developed until about 6 months or so after birth

Functions:
- Receives light
- Transmits light
- Converts light to visual energy

Central and peripheral retina compared.

Central retina close to the fovea is considerably thicker than peripheral retina. This is due to the increased packing density of photoreceptors, particularly the cones, and their associated bipolar and ganglion cells in central retina compared with peripheral retina. The Central retina is cone-dominated retina whereas peripheral retina is rod-dominated. Thus, in central retina the cones are closely spaced and the rods fewer in number between the cones

Macula lutea.

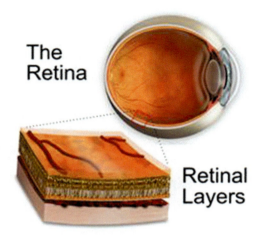

The Retina

Retinal Layers

This pigmentation is the reflection from yellow screening pigments, the xanthophyll carotenoids zeaxanthin and lutein (Balashov and Bernstein, 1998), present in the cone axons of the Henle fiber layer. The macula lutea is thought to act as a short wavelength filter, additional to that provided by the lens (Rodieck, 1973). As the fovea is the most essential part of the retina for human vision, protective mechanisms for avoiding bright light and especially ultraviolet irradiation damage are essential. The Cones form a concentrated area in the retina known as the fovea, which lies in the center of macula lutea. Damage to this area can severely reduce the ability to see directly ahead. Damage to rods results in night blindness but with retention of good visual acuity for straight-ahead objects.

The junction of the peripheral of the retina and the ciliary is called ora serrata. In the extreme periphery of the retina there are no cones and only a few rods. The retina is firmly attached to the choroid at the ora serrata. This is the reason that retinal detachments never extend beyond the ora serrata. The other site of firm attachment of the retina is at the circumference of the optic nerve. The posterior layer of the retina, called the pigment epithelium, is firmly secured to the choroid. Retinal detachment occurs as a result of cleavage between its anterior layers and posterior pigment layer.

Degenerative diseases of the human retina in related to Low Vision:
As well described in the above notes, the human retina is a thin, semitransparent, multilayered sheet of neural tissue that lines the inner aspect of the posterior two-thirds of the wall of the globe. If it's damaged, low vision or blindness may be the result. Some of the related eye disorders include:

- **Age related macular degeneration (AMD)** is a complex multifactorial progressive disease that generally affects people aged over 55 and is the leading cause of irreversible blindness in the developed world. Although the pathogenesis of AMD is still not cleared, many eye care specialists agreed that it's caused by degeneration of the Retinal Pigment Epithelium (RPE) due to oxidative stress which also lead to damage of the overlying photoreceptors (cones and rods).

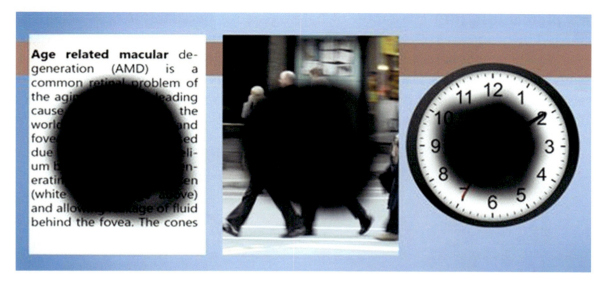

Age related macular degeneration (AMD) is a
common retinal problem of
the aging ... leading
cause ... the
world ... and
fove ... ed
due ... eli-
um ... en-
erati ... en
(white ... ove)
and allo ... age of fluid
behind the fovea. The cones

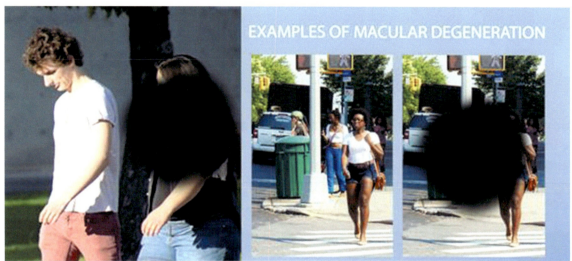

EXAMPLES OF MACULAR DEGENERATION

Glaucoma is a term used to describe a group of conditions having the common feature of an elevated intraocular pressure, resulting in loss of visual function. The loss of vision usually begins in the peripheral rather than the central field.

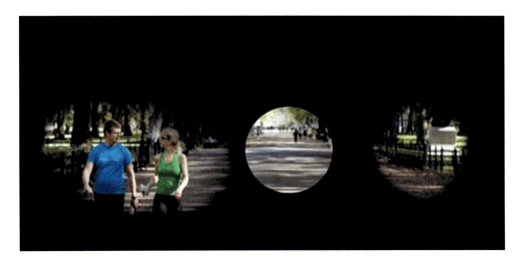

Retinitis pigmentosa (RP) is a group of heterogeneous hereditary retinal degenerations characterized by progressive dysfunction of the photoreceptors along with atrophy of several retinal layers. This nasty hereditary disease of the retina lead to progressive visual field loss, night blindness(nyctalopia), and abnormal ERG recording which often shows markedly reduced or absent retinal function. The occurrence of RP varies with age (noticeable in childhood, 3rd or 5th decade...etc. It is predominant in males.

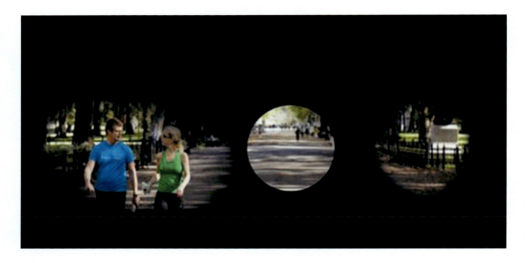

Diabetic retinopathy is a vascular complication of both type I (Insulin-dependent) and type II (Non-Insulin-dependent) diabetes mellitus. It occurs when small blood vessels in the eye stop feeding the retina which can lead to ischemia and subsequent neovascularization. With this condition, clients experience distorts vision, night blindness(nyctalopia), scattered blind spots or floaters in their field of vision and overall blurring vision...etc.

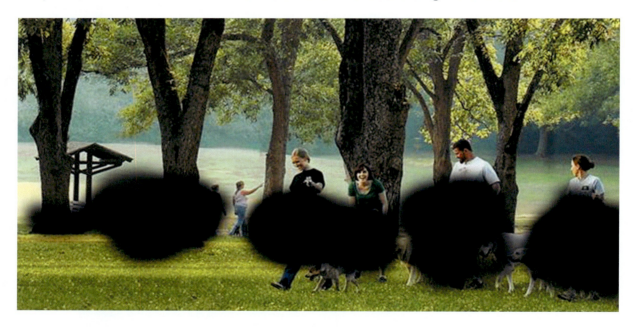

Laser treatment for stopping blood vessel proliferation and leakage of fluid into the retina, is the commonest treatment at present.

OPTIC NERVE HEAD

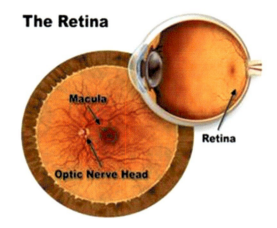

The Optic Nerve is a collection of 1 million nerve fibers. They are an extension of the last (of the 10) layers of the retina bundled like a cable of individual electrical wires

The optic nerve is:
- Formed by the nerve fiber layer of the retina
- There are 1 million optic nerve fibers
- The optic nerve exits the eye via that specialized portion of the sclera, the mesh-like lamina sclera cribosa
- The blind spot is where the optic nerve leaves the eye

The **function** of the optic nerve is to carry the nerve impulses from the eye (retina) to (ultimately) the visual cortex.

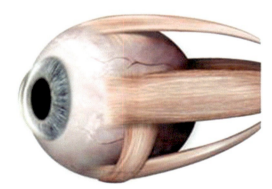

Side view of eye, extraocular muscles (70= inferior rectus muscle, 69 = lateral rectus muscle, 68 = superior rectus muscle).

THE PHYSIOLOGY OF VISION

How Human see?

Sight is considered as the sense in which the brain receives approximately 75% of its information. Sight is made possible by the eye, serving as a channel through which visual information is perceived. For an individual to see, there must be light.The perception of the visual stimulus occurs in several stages. The light first touches the thin veil of tears that coat the front of the eye. Behind this lubricating moisture is the window of the eye called **cornea**. Light will pass through this structure (cornea) which will help to focus the light (refractive power). The amount of light passing through the cornea will be determined by the size of the pupil. It then passes to a clean watery fluid called the **aqueous humor** which circulates throughout the front part of the eye to keep a constant pressure within the eye. Light will continue its way to the **pupil** which is a hole or opening in the colored part of the eye called the **Iris**. Depending on how much light there is, the Iris may contract or dilate, limiting or increasing the amount of light that gets deeper into the eye. Light then will go through the lens, the shape of which is adjusted by intraocular muscles to focus light on the retina. The **lens** changes shape to focus on light reflecting from near or distant objects. Finally, light passes through the layers of the **retina** to reach the photoreceptive layer of rods and cones. However, for light to be received unimpeded by the retina, the ocular structures above must be transparent. The outer segments of rods and cones transduce light energy from photons into membrane potentials. Then, the photo pigments in rods and cones absorb photons and this causes a conformational change in the molecular structure of these pigments. This molecular alteration causes sodium channels to close, which lead to hyperpolarization of membranes of the rods and cones and a reduction in the amount of neurotransmitter in the light and more neurotransmitter in the dark. Rods and cones have synaptic contacts on bipolar cells that project to ganglions cells. These photoreceptors on the retina travel along nerve fibers to a nerve bundle called the **optic nerve**, which exit's the back of the eye. The optic nerve will send the signal to the visual in the back of the brain (occipital area).

In summary, light reflected from object will enter the eye, focus then convert into electrochemical signals, which will deliver to the brain and then interpreted as an image.

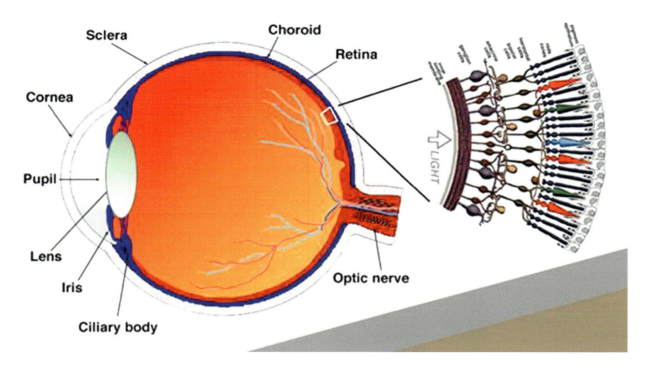

Rods and Cones

Diagram of rods and cones

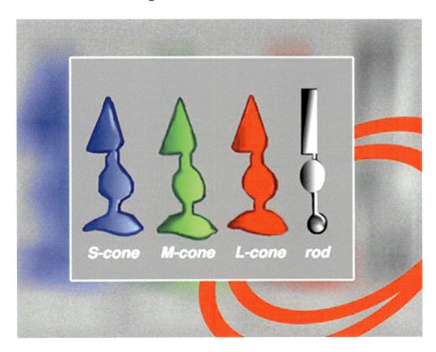

Rods and cones are specialized nerve cells. They contain an outer segment, which is sensitive to light, and an inner segment, which is like a typical axon or inner portion of a nerve cell.

Rods

The rods allow us to see at night and to perceive motion. The visual discrimination is of rods is not very high. They function in scotopic conditions (low illumination). There are about 100 to 125 million rods in the retina. Rods are in the peripheral retina. There are no rods in the macular area. Hundreds of rods connect (converge) through the bipolar and the other middle cells before connecting to a few ganglions. This allows our side vision to act as the travel vision. The rods function in scotopic conditions and provide vision in shades of gray.

Rods have an outer segment, nucleus and an inner segment. The outer segment consists of discs. These discs have a cell membrane and contain the visual pigment - rhodopsin. Rhodopsin is also commonly called "visual purple". Rhodopsin is a form of vitamin A. These discs are produced and discarded on a regular basis. The discs, which recycle every 7 days, are digested at the RPE. Problems with the regeneration of the discs are probably linked to the degenerative process in Retinitis pigmentosa. The absorption of light by the rhodopsin starts a chain reaction, which results in scotopic and travel vision.

Cones

Cones provide our detailed, color and phototropic (bright light) vision. There are approximately 6 to 8 million cones in the retina. Cones are the <u>only</u> photoreceptors in the foveola. There is a one-to-one connection of cones to ganglion cells in the retina. This is why the macular has such accurate and detailed vision. The cones are tightly packed together in the macular area. Cones are less light sensitive, requiring lighter to be stimulated.

Cones also consist of an outer segment, nucleus and inner segment. The visual pigment of the cones is contained in discs in the outer segment of the cones. Cones have three visual pigments:

- Erythrolabe: Red catching
- Chlorolabe: Green catching
- Cyanolabe: Blue catching

The combination of red, green and blue cones contributes to our perception of color.

Chapter 2:
Basic Optical Principles of the Eye and Refractive Disorders

First let us consider **the nature of light**:

Light and how it works is a fascinating and intricate topic. It is easier to comprehend using simplified models of light rays and wave fronts. Light is composed of many rays of light. A ray of light is a very thin beam, which travels in a straight line. A wave front is a surface, which is comprised of light rays, which left the initial source at the same time (like the sun for example). If light is traveling from a distance (20 feet or more away), it travels in parallel lines.

Reflection and Refraction:
When light hits a surface or a medium (of a different index of refraction) the light rays may be reflected or refracted. Parallel light rays traveling in air are refracted as they move through the cornea, aqueous, lens and vitreous (the pupil is merely a hole or aperture). The light rays come to a point of focus meet the surface of the cornea first, then the aqueous, lens and vitreous. The major refraction of lights happens at the cornea and lens. Light rays should come to a perfect point of focus in an eye without a refractive error (emmetropia).

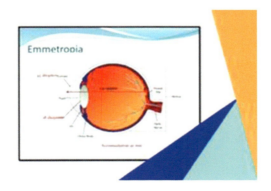

What is myopia and how is it corrected?

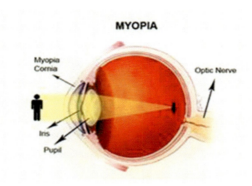

A condition in which the visual image is focused in front of the retina, resulting in a defective distance vision. The patient is near sighted and sees objects more clearly at near than distance. A concave negative (-) lens is used to correct this condition. The power of the lens is expressed in negative diopters.

What is hyperopia and how is it corrected?

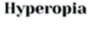
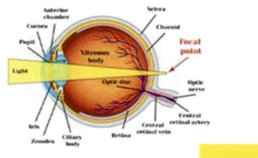

A condition in which the visual image is focused behind the retina, which may result in defective near vision. A convex () positive (+) lens is used to correct this condition. The power of the lens is expressed in diopters.

What is astigmatism and how is it corrected?

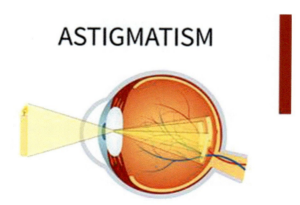

A condition cause by irregular curvature of the cornea and/or lens which prevents light rays from coming to a single point of focus on the retina. Instead, the light rays form image lines at different locations resulting in a blurred or distorted image. A cylindrical lens is used to correct this condition.

What is presbyopia and how is it corrected?

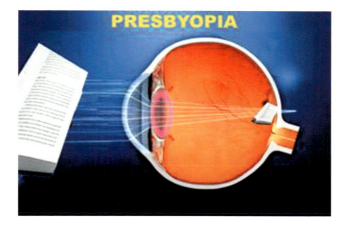

It refers to a condition in which there is a decrease in ability of the eye to accommodate. Accommodation is that action of the ciliary muscle which cause the lens to become more convex. In this situation, additional plus lens (more plus power) will be needed to correct it. The extra plus power will bend the light right from object at near. We loss this ability as we age.

An image is magnified with an object in front of a **<u>concave</u>** mirror

Emmetropia

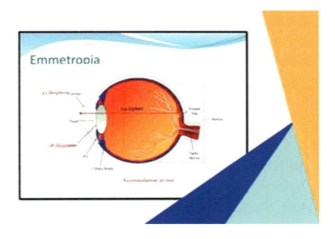

An emmetropic eye refracts (bends) light coming from a distance to a point of focus on the retina (when the eye is a state of rest). The emmetropic eye is considered to be a normal eye.

A few Examples of error of refraction:
With astigmatism, two differing powers or types of lenses are needed to bring the image to one point of focus on the retina. The lenses that are need involve both a sphere and a cylinder lens. This power is usually ground into the lenses. Please see demonstration below:

Compound Hyperopic Astigmatism (eye with hyperopia and astigmatism)
Prescription (RX)
+3:00 -.75 x 180 for example
Compound Myopic Astigmatism (eye with myopia and astigmatism)
Prescription (RX)
-4:00-1:00 X 90
-4:00 is the spherical lens and –1:00 is the cylinder. The cylinder is oriented at 90 degrees.

Magnification
Magnification is defined as the ratio of height of the image to the height of the object. This is also related to the image distance to the object distance. This is expressed in the formulas below

$$m = Hi/Ho = Di/Do$$

Note: m is magnification, Hi is the height of the image, Ho is the height of the object, Di is the image distance, Do is the object distance.

Note: a magnification of "1" (either minus or plus) means the image is equal to the same size as the original object.

However, is "m" being greater than "1" the image is bigger than the object. If the "m" is less than "1" then the image is smaller than the object. Whether or not the image is inverted or upright is related to being positive or negative. If the magnification value is positive the image will be upright. If the value of "m" is negative (compared to the object), the image will be inverted (again compared to the object).

The principle of Magnification is used in many devices used in low vision rehabilitation services (magnifiers and telescopes for example).

Knowledge of Optical and Non-Optical Equipment and Intervention Strategies:
Optical and Non-Optical devices are designed to improve visual performance in individuals with low vision or blindness, thus enabling academic and social adaptation and providing enrichment of daily living experiences.

Types of Devices:

Optical
When conventional lenses do not provide required visual range, aids that have optical properties capable of promoting better visual performance through lenses are indicated for the followings:

- Distance (telescope)
- Intermediate distance (tele microscope)
- Near (microscope)

Non-optical

Non-optical aids are visual aids that improve visual function without using magnified lenses. They include several adaptations, such as reading stands, supplemental lighting, absorptive sunglasses, typoscopes, and tactile locator dots etc... They enhance visual function by:

- Linear magnification (magnification brought about by enlarging the object itself). $M_s =$ S/S' M_s = Relative size magnification, S = Enlarged print size and S' = Size of the original print

Proper lighting is critical for good vision. As we age, a person age 65 or older probably needs 15 times as much light to read as does a 10-year-old. And importantly, a person with low vision may need three times as much light to read as a person their age who does not have a vision loss. Lighting necessity varies for every individual and depends on the diagnosis and extent of pathology. Diseases such as aniridia, achromatopsia, and albinism require low-level lighting; glaucoma, retinitis pigmentosa, optic atrophy, and nuclear cataract require high illumination. A typoscope, caps or visors, side shields, and/or polarizing lenses should be prescribed to control the reflection of light. A typoscope can also be used as a guide to be reading, writing, and signature in cases of large defects of visual field. A person who has had a stroke and resultant hemianopia can benefit from a typoscope when reading.

Light-filtering lenses are useful and frequently prescribed. They should filter ultraviolet radiation below 400 nm, minimizing the loss of VA and color discrimination. It is important to consider comfort; protection from ultraviolet, infrared, and visible light; increased contrast; and glare reduction.

Several factors should be considered when choosing a filter: lens color, photo-chromaticity, optical density, polarization, and spectrum of protection. The filters can be adapted in glasses, clip-ons, or contact lenses.

Different filters can be prescribed for different situations, paying close attention to the goals to be achieved, levels of lighting, cost, and especially the individual preference.

Enhanced contrast (Absorptive lenses in yellow for low-light environments and amber for more intense lighting are good prescription options. Absorptive sunglasses help filter out bothersome glare and harmful light rays. Most sunglasses now block out ultraviolet light. However, to block out "blue" light, which causes concern for macular degeneration and other eye conditions, sunglasses need to have some amount of yellow in them. The colors of sunglasses that contain some yellow and block out blue light are amber, orange, amber/orange combination, plum, and yellow. Grey and green-grey colored sunglasses do not block out any blue light. Grey and green-grey sunglasses also do not provide as good contrast as do amber, orange, plum, and yellow.

It is also important to support daily activities with aids such as black felt-tipped pen, bold lines, and contrasting colors).

- Reduction of glare
- Improving physical comfort: For a better acceptance and adaptation to the optical aid, physical comfort is key. An inclined board set at a 45-degree angle can be of help.

Electronic

Electronic devices include video magnifier systems, closed-circuit televisions, Bluetooth connections to smart projectors, large-print computer programs such as Zoom Text, screen readers such as Virtual Vision and Jaws, and computer tablets.

It is important to consider that with VA of 20/50 (0.5 logMar) the child can perform most of the daily tasks. In this way, the Kestenbaum rule can be applied, in which the magnification is given by the inverse of the VA in diopters (A = 1/VA). To achieve the power of hand or stand magnifiers and telescopes: divide the value found in diopters by 4 (unit of magnification), for example:

VA = 20/200
A = 200/20 = 10 D/4 = 2.5X

VA = 20/160, desiring to achieve 20/20
A = 160/20 = 8X

Select the aid according to the characteristics of the device: the needs, goals, motivations, and clinical aspects of the patient. Remember that the lighting and reading conditions in client home are very different from those in a specially designed low vision clinic or office. Like any other skill, learning to read with a low vision device requires regular practice over many weeks.

Chapter 3:
Common Disorders and Diseases of the Eye
(Mostly Encountered in Low Vision)

SIGNS AND SYMPTOMS OF EYE DISEASE

This section will provide information on common signs and symptoms of vision problems. This information should alert you to ocular emergencies and serious eye diseases. Behavior and symptoms specific to children is found at the end of the chapter.

ONSET OF VISION PROLEM

One important way to consider vision problems or losses is by their mode of onset. The modes are: acute, gradual, and transient.

Acute vision losses involve a rapid onset of change in visual performance. An acute vision loss is often an ocular emergency. True ocular emergencies include retinal detachments, central retinal artery or central retinal vein occlusions.

Gradual or slow onset of visual loss typically means the problem was chronic or long-standing in nature. A classic condition exhibiting slow vision loss is senile cataracts.

A **transient vision** loss means the vision change is temporary. It can be a chronic or acute vision problem. It is not necessarily an emergency. Asthenopia is blurry vision from eye fatigue such a prolonged reading. This chronic condition usually indicates a need for prescription change or visual training for an eye muscle imbalance.

Whereas transient ischemic attack (T.I.A.) is a serious acute loss of vision caused by a temporary blockage of the central retinal artery. It is often a precursor to an impending stroke. The underlying etiology (cause) is vascular disease.

ASTHENOPIA (eye fatigue)

If a patient complains of strain or fatigue while or after performing visual tasks, one should investigate the presence of a muscle imbalance (causing problems with focusing and/or directing the eyes), double vision (diplopia) when reading or a refractive change (especially for tasks at near).

CURTAINS

A person who is experiencing a retinal detachment may report seeing curtains being drawn down or a glass being filled up with ink. Retinal detachments are another true ocular emergency. The retina is actually only attached to the ora serrata (front-most part of the retina) and the optic nerve head. The rest of the retina lies against the choroid. The retinal detaches (or separates) there is a break from its nutritional sources. Permanent vision loss occurs after a short period of time.

Curtains coming down could also be a sign of an ophthalmic migraine. Ophthalmic migraines occur more in woman then men. They often start in the third decade of life. The symptoms may or may not be accompanied by a headache. There can be a sudden vision loss or perception of colors or bizarre visual patterns. There is nothing wrong with the eyes with an ophthalmic migraine. The first time the person has an attack it may have similar signs of a retinal detachment. With time, the person will often learn the pattern of an impending migraine.

DIPLOPIA (Double Vision)

If a patient complains of double vision, one must first ascertain if the diplopia is in one or both eyes.

Monocular diplopia is that which occurs with one eye; it could possibly indicate the presence of a cataract.

Monocular diplopia is not true diplopia. Binocular diplopia (that which occurs with both eyes open) it is true diplopia. Diplopia of sudden onset in an elderly individual is a muscle imbalance that could be clue to an aneurysm, diabetes, arteriosclerosis, or a cerebrovascular accident (CVA).

FLASHES OF LIGHT

Flashes of light followed by spots may indicate a retinal or vitreal detachment or perhaps a retinal tear. A patient may also report seeing streaks of lightening or another visual disturbance.

Vitreous detachment is seen in about 60% of elderly persons. It presents like a retinal detachment and should be treated like an ocular emergency until it is determined otherwise. Vitreal detachments are followed closely for about one month since they can sometimes lead to a retinal detachment. Remember, the vitreous is attached to the retina at the ora serrata, macular and the optic nerve head.

Again, migraine headache can also present with similar signs as a retinal detachment.

HALOS

Halos or rings around streetlights during the night (or dim illumination) can mean there is edema (fluid) in the cornea. This could be an indication of glaucoma or swelling of the cornea from a contact lens over wear. Another cause of halos is corneal degeneration.

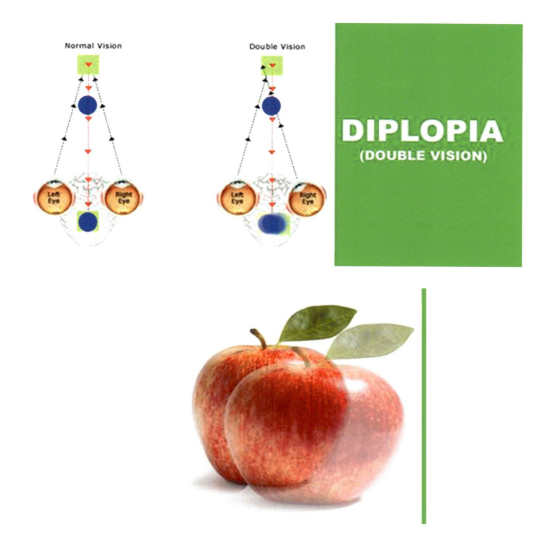

ITCHING AND BURNING

Itching and burning was discussed under sandy, gritty feeling in the eye. Again, itchiness is a classic symptom for an allergic reaction. Burning may accompany a viral insult to the eye.

NIGHT BLINDNESS (Nyctalopia)

Nyctalopia is decreased visual function/ability when going from a performance in dim illumination (such as the night) or other scotopic conditions. It is called night blindness since it usually occurs most frequently at nighttime.

Night blindness may be caused by a vitamin A deficiency. It may also indicate the earlier stages of a very serious progressive inherited disorder - retinitis pigmentosa (RP). Vitamin A is needed to form the visual pigment used by rods in the "seeing" process. Other retinal degenerative conditions are characterized by night blindness.

PHOTOPHOBIA

An acute or sudden sensitivity to bright lights may indicate the presence of an iritis or a keratitis (inflammation of the iris and cornea respectively). A posterior uveitis is an inflammation of the choroid (the middle coat of the eye, it supports the retina). An anterior Uveitis is an inflammation of the ciliary body and/or and iris of the eye. A keratitis can lead to uveitis. Persons will blue eyes; misshapen pupil and or Albinism may chronically suffer from of photophobia (there is a lack of light control in the iritis).

SANDY FEELING

Persons complaining of a gritty, sandy feeling in the eye may have conjunctivitis (inflammation of the conjunctiva), dry eye, or a corneal abrasion due to foreign body or contact lens over wear. Conjunctivitis is usually from allergies if there is itchiness, bacterial if it fells sandy and viral if it is burn and teary.

Dry eyes are usually caused by a reduction in the quality of the tears as we age or are related to arthritis. Most patients present with watery eyes. This is caused by the dryness and constant irritation of the cornea. These tears are not the type that provides nutrition and lubrication to the cornea. Corneal abrasion or a foreign body/object in the cornea causes great pain, blurry vision and excessive tearing.

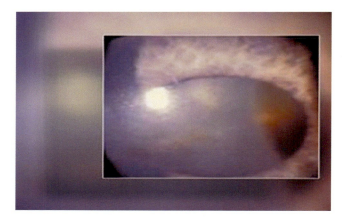

SPOTS/FLOATERS

Spots and floaters in the eye can be very normal. Some people have floaters because the temporary blood vessel system (Hyaloid), which nourishes the prenatal eye, does not fully disappear and remnants (debris) are left behind. Sometimes older adults develop floaters as the vitreous ages. It could also indicate diabetes and/or possible retinal tears or detachments (if accompanied by a loss of vision or visual field loss).

As the eye ages, the vitreous liquefies and may detach from the retina and optic nerve head (remember - the vitreous is the gel -like substance in the large chamber in the back of the eye).

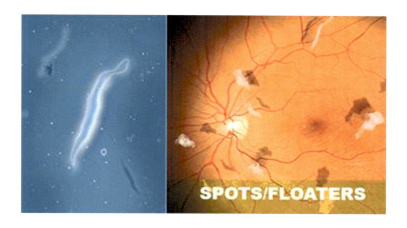

TENDERNESS

If a person complains of pain and soreness of the eyes, one must consider the possibility of external and internal ocular inflammations as well as narrow angle glaucoma. Patients with internal ocular inflammations like, as cellulitis will present with pain, redness and swelling of the lids. Intraocular inflammations such as an anterior uveitis would present as a sore, uncomfortable eye with a pinpoint pupil. Narrow angle glaucoma is characterized by severe brow pain, nausea and perhaps vomiting. The patient may report seeing halos around lights. The cornea may appear very cloudy and the vision will be reduced. The person will be extremely uncomfortable.

OCULAR ABBREVIATIONS:

A	Anterior
AC	Anterior Chamber
C	with spectacles (it is a little "c")
AS	Arteriolar Sclerosis
A/V	Artery to vein ratio
ARM	Age related maculopathy
BID	Twice a day
BVA	Best visual acuity
CC	Chief complaint
C/D	Cup to disc ration
CF	Counts fingers
COAG	Chronic Open Angle Glaucoma
CRA	Central retinal artery
CRV	Central retinal vein
CVA	Cerebral vascular accident (AKA stroke)
D	Lens Diopters
DR	Diabetic Retinopathy
HR	Hypertensive Retinopathy
HBP/HTN	High blood pressure/Hypertension

DX	Diagnosis
E	Esophoria
EOM	Extraocular muscles
ET	Esotropia
EV	Eccentric viewing
EX	Examination
FT	Flat top (type of bifocal lens)
FX	Findings
HA	Headache
HM	Hand motion
HX	History
IN	Inferior temporal
IOP	Intraocular pressure
IT	Inferior temporal
KP	Keratic Precipitate
LP	Light perception
NLP	No light perception
NPC	Near point of convergence
OD	Right eye also Doctor of Optometry
ODM	Ophthalmo-dynamometry
OKN	Optokinetic nystagmus
OS	Left eye
OU	Both eyes
P	Posterior
PD	Pupillary distance
PERRLA	Pupils equal round and respond to light and accommodation
PH	Pinhole
PRS	As needed
PSC	Posterior subcapsular cataract
PVD	Posterior vitreous detachment
PX	Prognosis
QD	Once a day
QID	Four times a day
RLF	Retrolental fibroplasia
R/O	Rule out
ROP	Retinopathy of prematurity
RP	Retinitis Pigmentosa
RTC	Return to clinic
RX	Prescription

S	without spectacles (little "s")
SLEx	Slit lamp exam
SMD	Senile macular degeneration
SN	Superior nasal
ST	Superior temporal
SX	Symptoms
Tap	Tonometry by applanation method
TID	Three times a day
TF	Trial frame
TX	Treatment
VA	Visual Acuity
VF	Visual Field
XT	Exotropia
W	Patient wears spectacles
WNL	Within normal limits
W/O	Without
X	Exophoria
XT	Exotropia
(+)	Plus lens
(-)	Minus lens

COMMON EYE DISEASES AND FUNCTIONAL IMPLICATIONS:
PART A - OVERALL DECREASED OR BLURRED VISION

Albinism
With this congenital condition, there is a lack of the pigment melanin in the body and/or eye. The patient has white skin, hair, pale fundus and pink appearing irides in complete systemic form. There is a normal coloring of hair, skin and irides in ocular form (though they tend to be fair). Eye color can range from very light blue to brown and may change with age.

Common functional problems:
- High refractive error and astigmatism
- Nystagmus
- Photophobia
- Extreme glare issues
- Reduced VA (about 20/200 due to underdeveloped macular)
- Children would have difficulty reading

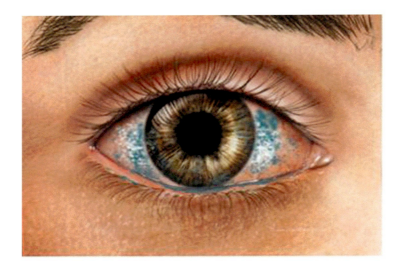

Individuals with albinism often have pale blue eyes and white eyelashes

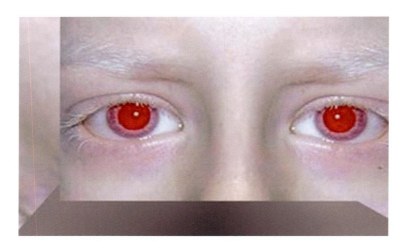

Albino eyes will appear very red when a light is shown into them.

Management Strategies:
- Magnification
- Good contrast, bold, high contrast magic markers
- Good refraction and prescriptive glasses
- Diffuse light from behind
- Glare reduction
- Light control (absorptive lenses, sunglasses, visors and shades)
- Frequent rest periods during close work

Amblyopia

Also known as **lazy eye.** Reduce visual in one eye is due to a strabismus (squint), uncorrected refractive error, or some type of media opacity (cornea or lens). The vision in the amblyopic eye does not develop optimally. Treatment is to patch the better seeing eye and performing visual training exercises with the lazy eye. Results vary but are a better prognosis exists if this therapy is done on a young child.

Common Functional Problems:
If the acuity is greater than 2-3 lines:
- Monocular vision
- Poor depth perception
- Glare problems.
- Possible eye fatigue at near
- Loss of place while reading.

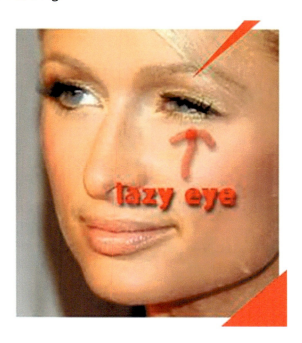

Management Strategies:
- If problems with near work - 15 minutes of rest for every hour of close work
- Consider rearranging student's seat to favor best eye
- Glare reduction
- Teach environmental cues for depth perception

Aniridia
In this congenital condition, there is a lack of visible iris. Light control to the back of the eye is poor because of the abnormal shaped pupil (extremely large). There are major issues with photophobia. This iris stumps often interfere with outflow of aqueous and glaucoma results. There is often a cataract accompanying aniridia. Vision loss with aniridia is a result of the accompanying glaucoma and cataract.

Common Functional Problems:
- Photophobia
- Glare
- Poor light adaptation

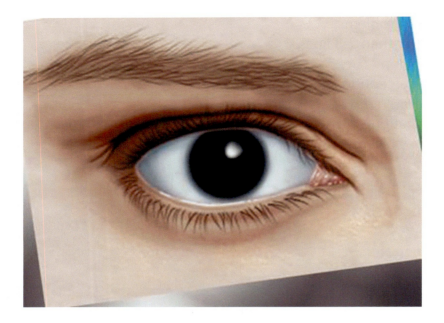

Management Strategies:
- Glare control- contact lens with artificial pupil, sunglasses, visors and absorptive lenses (with side shields)
- Magnification for any reduced VA
- Adjust lighting to dim illumination

Aphakia
No lens if the eye. There is often a cataract (opacity/cloudiness of the lens)
Common Functional Problems:
- Depth perception if monocular
- No accommodation

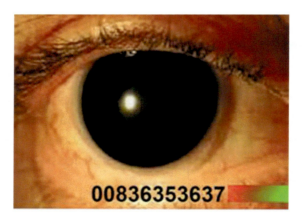

Management Strategies:
- Good lighting (gooseneck or adjustable lamps are good for close work)
- Magnification
- Good contrast
- Glare control (sunglasses and visor, indoors if necessary)
- Glasses or contacts should be worn for classroom work

Cataracts

Cataracts are an opacity or cloudiness of the lens of the eye. Light is not able to pass through the lens to the back of the eye to a normal degree. The denser the cataract, the less light that is transmitted to the retina. The visual fields plot normal.

Common Functional Problems:
- Constricted pupil (age or medication)
- Blurred vision
- Crossed eye (strabismus) if congenital in one eye
- Peripheral field distortion (from the aphakic lenses)
- Inability to accommodate
- Poor depth perception
- Photophobia,
- Glare

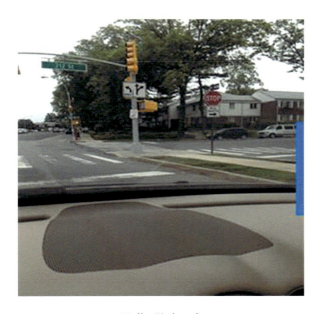

(Fully Sighted)

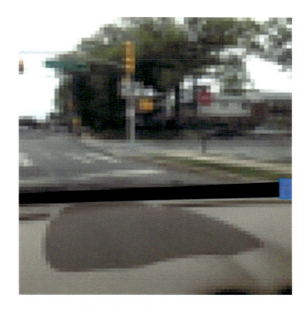

(Blur View from someone diagnosed with cataract)

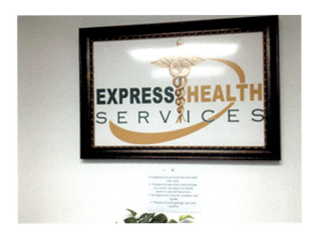

(Fully Sighted)

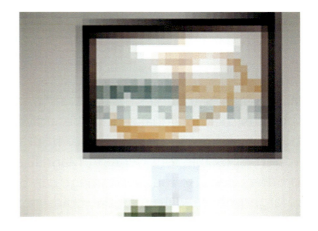

Management Strategies:
- After surgery, children need lenses or contact lenses (almost all adults and some children will get an IOL implant)
- Because the eye cannot accommodate without the lens, students should bring material close to the eye will magnify the image,
- Lighting is best behind the client on the side of the good eye
- Reduce glare by use of filters, tints, and sun lenses
- If cataracts are not removed bright light is needed
- Adjustable gooseneck lighting is advised
- Wear glasses or contact lenses to replace power of removed lens
- Clients will need to rest their eyes
- Nonoptical devises, such as large-print reading material, bold-line writing paper, and a typoscope may be helpful

Corneal Dystrophy

A group of inherited conditions that result in mild to major loss of transparency of the cornea. The visual acuity is mild to severe depending on the area of the cornea affecting and denseness of the opacification. The central and peripheral fields plot normal.

Common Functional Problems:
- Decreased vision
- Glare problems
- Illumination issues (not enough light)

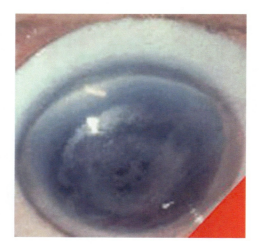

Management Strategies:
This must be individualized to the individual. It would depend on the extent of the opacity, location and depth of the opacity from the dystrophy. Illumination, print size, magnification would be possible consideration. Magnification may be beneficial to some clients but detrimental to others because the ghost image can become magnified as well. Non optical systems, such as large-print reading material, bold-line writing paper, and typoscope, may be helpful.

Part B-MIXED AND OTHER VISION LOSSES

Optic Atrophy
The optic nerve is a bundle of nerve fibers that carry images from your retina to your brain. Each fiber carries a part of the visual information to the brain. If these nerve fibers become damaged, the brain doesn't receive all this vision information and sight becomes blurred. Optic atrophy means the loss of some or most of the nerve fibers in the optic nerve. The effects range from visual change to severe visual loss.

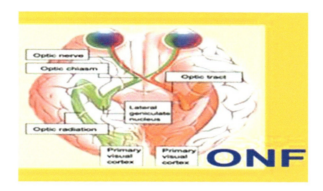

Optic nerve fibers from each eye meet and connect at the chiasm.
Damage to the optic nerve in front of the chiasm only affects that one eye.

Optic atrophy is not a disease, but rather a sign of a potentially more serious condition. Optic nerve atrophy is a result of many ocular and systemic disease as well as external factors such as toxins or trauma. It is difficult to predict the progression of optic nerve atrophy. The coloration changes (pallor of the disc) occur after the atrophy has happened.

Anatomy affected - the last layer of the retina is the nerve fiber layer. The nerve fibers (axons of the ganglion cells of the retina) gather from the ENTIRE retina and exit each eye as the optic nerve. Therefore, the possibilities to visual acuity and visual field loss are endless. Complete optic atrophy results in total blindness. Generally, client has the following signs and symptoms:
- Blurred vision
- Abnormal side vision
- Abnormal color vision, sluggish pupillary response to light, photophobia, and possible nystagmus
- Decreased brightness in one eye relative to the other (A reduction in sharpness of vision)

Please be advised that the symptoms described above may not necessarily mean that you have optic atrophy. However, if your clients experience one or more of these symptoms, you should advise them to contact their Eye care Specialist for a complete exam.

Common Physiological Problems:
- Scotoma (different locations)
- Decreased VA
- In general, teachers should avoid use of busy patterns and backgrounds

- Modify educational performance to visual problem experienced (central scotoma versus field constriction - see above conditions)
- For congenital atrophy consider vision stimulation activities

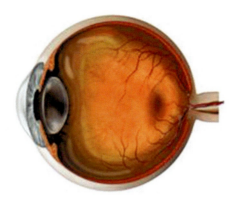

Management Strategies:
Remediation would correspond to the type of client's functional problem (field enhancement and mobility training for tunnel vision, magnification for reduced vision, lighting adaptation for glare control and so on). Excessive lighting should be avoided. Sun lenses, tints, and filters may help to eliminate glare, both indoors and outdoors. Non optical systems, such as large-print reading material, bold-line writing paper, and typoscope, may be helpful. Genetic counseling will also be very helpful for clients diagnosed with hetero-degenerative forms of optic atrophy.

Diabetic Retinopathy
This is a complication from long-term Diabetes. This is another condition where damage can occur in a variety of ways. (See above note). In diabetic retinopathy, the supporting cells of the retinal capillaries (pericytes or small blood vessels) die off, thereby weakening the capillary wall and allowing formation of microaneurysms. With progression, there will be a breakdown of the blood-retina barrier, which will allow blood constituents to leak or rupture into the retina. The leak of fluid in the retina may affect not only the macula, but also the vitreous (the clear, gel like substance that fills the interior of the eye). Most of the times, this leaking fluid distorts client's visions. This explains the overall blurring or scattered blind spots presented by individuals with this condition. (See picture below).

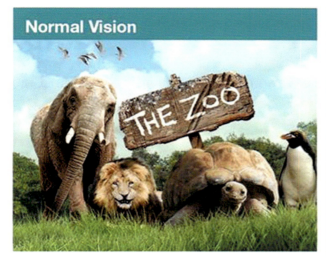

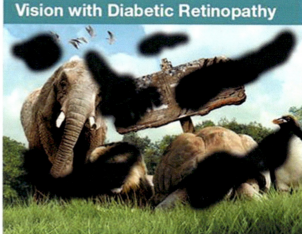

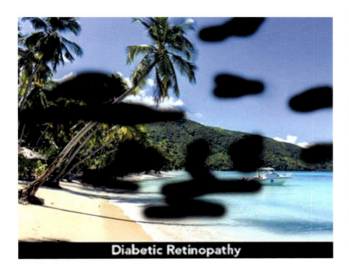

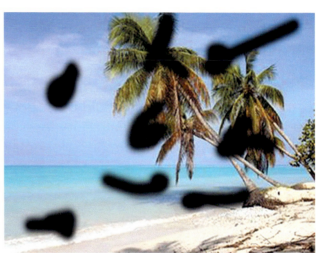

Scattered blind spot/blurring

Common Functional Problems:
This would depend on the part or parts of the eye affected (retinal detachment, hemorrhage in macular area, vitreal hemorrhage etc.) but may include:

- Loss of vision
- Fluctuation vision with uncontrolled blood sugar
- Floaters in the vitreous (seen as spots or spider webs)
- Retinal detachment
- Retinal hemorrhages
- Macular edema, macular hemorrhages
- Visual field defects
- Reduced color vision
- Scotoma (s)

Management Strategies:

Remediation of problems would relate to area affected however that may include:

- Magnification
- Good lighting
- Enhance contrast for classroom and home environment (for color vision problems), high contrast markers for schoolwork
- Eccentric viewing if needed
- Field enhancement if needed
- Diet and stress affect blood sugars – keep sugars at recommended levels
- Stress management
- Poor diet can affect clarity of thinking – improve diet

Coloboma

Coloboma is a congenital malformation of one or both eyes, in which there is a gap (notch, cleft) or hole in one of the multiple structures of the eye. So, during gestation, there is a defect in the closure of the embryonic cleft. The most typical missing tissue (hole) is the iris, retina and sometimes optic nerve (usually at the six o'clock position).

If there were a hole in the retina, there would be a corresponding scotoma. Again, if it were a six o'clock coloboma, there would be a superior defect (the person would tend to hit his/her head). The most serious visual acuity loses, and visual field losses occur with an optic nerve coloboma. The visual problems in Coloboma depends on which part of the eye is affected and how extensive it is.

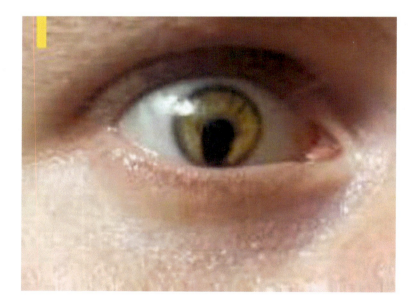

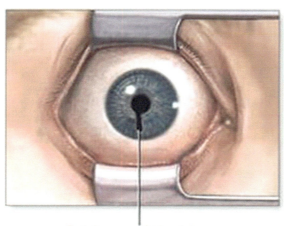

Coloboma of the iris

Common Functional Problems:
- Photophobia
- Nystagmus
- Scotoma
- Field loss
- Decreased acuity
- Possibly cataracts

Management Strategies:
- Cosmetic contact lenses (they have an artificial pupil)
- Light control – eyeglasses, eye shade (for iris coloboma). Client may function better in environment with reduced illumination
- Magnification if there is reduced acuity
- Bold markers for schoolwork
- Typoscopes may help with finding sentences, data
- Instruct how to scan the daily living environment to avoid superior obstructions.

Coloboma – Associated Syndromes:
1. Trisomy 13 (Patau's syndrome). Coloboma is associated with this chromosomal disorder in almost 100% of cases.
2. Aicardi's Syndrome. Coloboma and gray optic disk coloration are fundus finding in this case.
3. Goldenhar's syndrome or oculoauriculovertebral dysplasia
4. CHARGE. Coloboma, Heart disease, Atresia choanae, Retarded growth, Genital hypoplasia, and

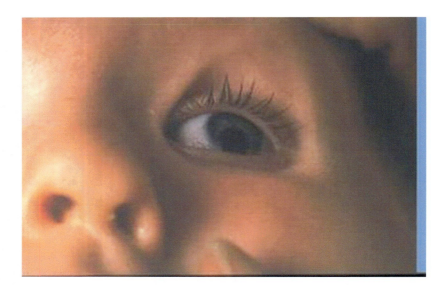

Coloboma and CHARGE association.

Retinoblastoma - Very serious tumor of childhood.

Retinoblastoma (Rb) is a rare form of cancer that rapidly develops from the immature cells of a retina, the light-detecting tissue of the eye. It is the most common malignant cancer of the eye in children, and it is almost always found in young children.

Common Functional Problems:
- Problems with depth perception if one eye was enucleated.
- The first sign of this disease may be white pupil (an abnormal appearance of the retina as viewed through the pupil, the medical term for which is leukocoria, also known as amaurotic cat's eye reflex) or turned eye
- Poor depth perception (curbs, stairs) A child with leukocoria due to retinoblastoma in the left eye

Management Strategies:
- Prosthetic eye
- Low vision devices and strategies if there is vision in remaining eyeOther diseases, which vary in terms of visual acuity deficit and/or field loss, include Hypertensive Retinopathy, Toxoplasmosis, Syphilis, HIV and Histoplasmosis to name a few.

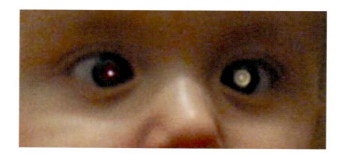

C-ANTERIOR SEGMENT EYE DISEASE EYESLIDS:

Eyelids
This is delicate **tissue** that **swells** easily. **It is** well-innervated and rich in **blood supply** (many fluids can pour into the eyelids). So, it is **very exposed** to the external environment.

1. **Hordeolum (stye)** - is a localized **acute** (quick onset) inflammation of lid glands.

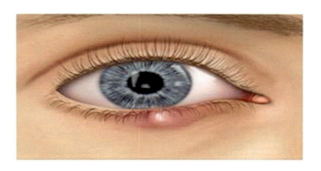

In the above image, there is a red area on the lower lid, it is a stye.

Usually patient presents with:
- Focalized tenderness (the pain is very local to the site of the blocked gland)
- **Lid swelling at /near the site of the gland inflammation**
- Possible pustule that point towards the sclera or the air (it looks like a white head of a pimple)

Treatment and management:
- Hot compresses (this dilates the blood vessels bringing healing cells to the area)
- Local topical antibiotics may be needed

Chalazion – is a **chronic** inflammation of the lid gland (it becomes clogged over a gradual period of time).

The patient presents with:
- a non-tender lump within eye (it may be larger than a stye)

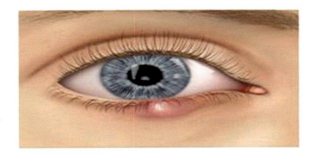

There is a large red lump on the middle of the upper lid, it is the chalazion.

Treatment and management:
- Hot compresses may be used but may not heal the chalazion
- In-office surgical removal may be needed if desired (cosmetically)

Blepharitis - is an inflammation of eyelid margins (edge of the eyelids where lashes insert)

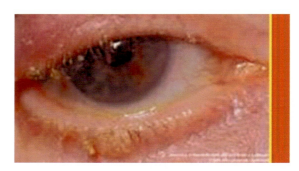

Types:
- Acute ulcerative/ bacterial
- Seborrheic/dandruff (dry skins falls from the head or scalp onto the lashes which serves as a nest and breeding ground for bacteria)

The patient presents with an irritation of the eyelid with debris or stickiness

Treatment and management:
- Good hygiene (wash eyelid, and scalp with baby shampoo for the seborrheic type)
- Topical antibiotic as indicated for the bacterial type

Note: children who have recurring Blepharitis and do not have dandruff of the scalp may be uncorrected hyperopes. Uncorrected hyperopes have eyestrain and tend to rub their eye a lot, causing a staphylococcus infection of the lid margins (Blepharitis).

Allergic reactions - in and around the lids are either an:
- Immediate allergic response called "The Wet Look", watery
- Delayed allergy usually because of a contact dermatitis; It is called "The Dry Look", scabbed and cracked skin

Usually patient presents with itchiness, which is classic for allergic reactions, arteries dilate and bring in histamines which itch, the lids feel irritated.

The treatment consists of:
- Identifying the allergen if possible and remove/disuse
- Using cold compresses on the affected area
- Using of local and systemic anti-inflammatories

Ecchymosis (black eye) – is a seepage of blood within lid tissue caused by trauma. The patient presents with black and blue discoloration and eyelid swelling

The treatment is:
- Cold compresses followed by warm compresses
- X-ray in case of orbital fracture (this can cause trapdoor fracture or muscle or nerve that innervate the EO muscles or create a passageway from the eye to the sinuses, very dangerous if there is a sinus infection and bacterial material is transmitted to the back of the eye)
- Eye examination to rule out ocular damage such as a tear to the root of the iris

Ptosis - is a drooping of the upper lid(s).

The patient present with monocular (one eye) or binocular (both eyes) ptosis. It may be a problem with the muscle itself (mechanical) or the nerve. Ptosis may be congenital or acquired in nature.

The treatment is:
- First rule out a pathology which must be dealt with (i.e., tumor pressing on nerve which lifts/open the lid)
- Fitting and use of a ptosis crutch – wire customized to insert into the fold of the eyelid with a spring, all of which is inserted discretely into the temple of a pair of spectacles. When the person closes the eye, the spring opens it back up.
- Surgical correction

NOTE: In an older individual, one can tell the whether a ptosis was congenital or acquired by merely looking at the lids without a history of the condition. The reason is with a congenital ptosis, there is not a lid fold (wrinkle) is the following. Lid folds develop from the eye being open (over time).

CONJUNCTIVA
The conjunctiva is thin layer of tissue embedded with blood vessels. It covers the sclera and end at the limbus of the cornea.

The conjunctiva's response to inflammation includes:
- Redness (also referred to as injection)
- Production of a discharge (watery, pussy or mucoid (whitish)
- Tissue changes like swelling/enlargement (chemosis)

Conjunctivitis (commonly known as pink eye) is the inflammation of the conjunctiva due to infection or irritation. The "red eye".

The conjunctiva is red and watery (depicted) in image below.

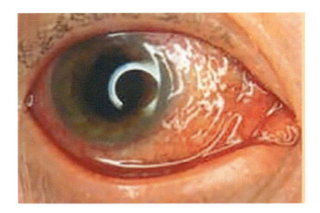

The patient presents with one of the following:
- **<u>Bacterial conjunctivitis</u>**: with redness, a **pussy** (yellowish) discharge and the patient reports having **gritty, sandy** or foreign body sensation. The treatment is topical eye drops
- **<u>Viral conjunctivitis</u>**: with redness, **teary** discharge, **burning** sensation. The treatment is time, until the virus runs its course, comfort drops, or cold compresses may make the patient "feel" better.
- **<u>Allergic conjunctivitis</u>**: redness, **mucous** discharge and **itching.** Treatment involves removal of allergen (if possible), antihistamine, ocular decongestants and cold compresses to constrict the blood vessels and limit the allergic response.
- **<u>Pinguecula</u>** - is fatty tissue which builds up in the conjunctiva, typically in the inner segment (canthus) or outer segment of the sclera.

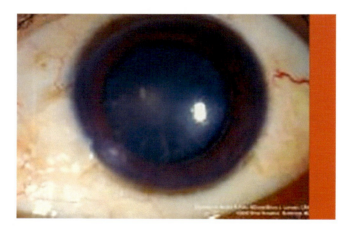

Pinquecula image.

Generally, patients notice the pinquecula when they have injected eyes or are looking intently and close up at their eyes after a new contact lens fitting. It may also be noted during a routine examination.

Because it is a benign tissue, no treatment is needed.

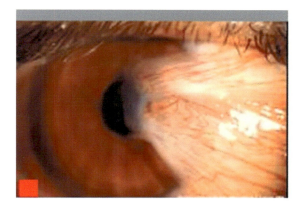

Pterygium – It's elastic tissue overgrowth from the conjunctiva onto the cornea (it is a pinguecula, which starts to grow towards the cornea). The image below is of a pterygium. It looks like a big wedge of tissue covering and approaching the right side of the cornea; it has its own blood vessels. Pterygia are noted often in patients with excessive outdoor exposure (ultraviolet light rays may cause the pinguecula tissue to grow).

Usually they stop growing by themselves (self-limiting); surgery is indicated when a good portion of the cornea is covered.

Subconjunctival hemorrhage is broken blood vessel beneath the conjunctiva. Usually the area of hemorrhage come to our practice due to the following conditions:
- Trauma
- Coughing, straining, vomiting
- Idiopathic in elderly patient

A subconjunctival hemorrhage is quite dramatic looking. The blood is very red and often covers the entire sclera in the inner or outer canthus of the eye.

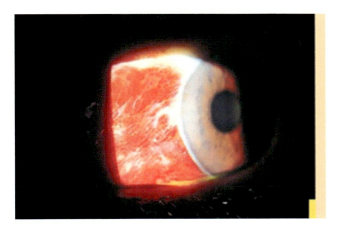

The left side of the above image shows the large very red area of hemorrhage, it stops just at the margin of the cornea.

The treatment is to be supportive and reassure the patient that everything is fine. They self-resolve in about seven days.

Conjunctival foreign body

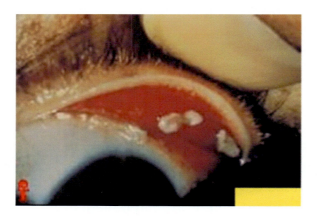

Conjunctival foreign body - a small foreign object (dust, dirt, splinter, glass etc.) is lodged on the conjunctiva (mucous membrane). The upper part of the image shows the white foreign body imbedded in the conjunctiva lining the lid. The patient presents with irritation and tearing.

The treatment is removal of foreign body in the office, usually with a wet swab or small hand instrument.

Cornea

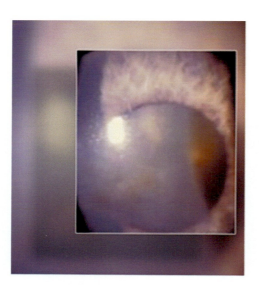

Since the Cornea represents the first ocular structure in the visual pathway, any conditions that affect it can be very serious due to the potential to disrupt its transparency.

Dry eye (keratitis sicca or keratoconjunctivitis sicca (KCS) - Corneal irritation due to inadequate or poor-quality tears. Dry eye may develop with age. Generally, client diagnosed with this condition presents with a gritty, sandy sensation in the eye. Chronic dry eye makes the cornea more susceptible to corneal infections.

The tear glands (lacrimal glands), located above each eyeball, continuously supply tear fluid that's wiped across the surface of your eye each time you blink your eyes. Excess fluid drains through the tear ducts into the nose.

Treatment may involve:
- Use of artificial tears during the day
- Use of a more viscous ointment in the eyes at night
- Use of lacrimal plugs (to keep the tears in the cornea longer)
- Blink training if their blink reflex has decreased (seen in the elderly)

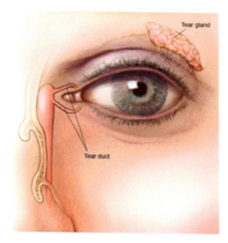

<u>Corneal abrasions</u> - a loss of corneal epithelium due to trauma (or contact lens over wear). The patient presents with pain, tearing, light sensitivity. They are extremely uncomfortable.

The treatment is:
- Pressure patching (this immobilizes the lids so the normal blinking of the eyes cannot rub the abraded cornea. Remember the cornea has the 2nd highest number of nerves/ tissues making it very painful when injured.
- Antibiotic ointment before patching to prevent infection.

<u>Keratitis:</u> An inflammation and infection of the cornea, which is due to any number of causes. Keratitis is sometimes caused by an infection involving bacteria, viruses, fungi or parasites. Noninfectious keratitis can be caused by a minor injury, wearing your contact lenses too long or other noninfectious diseases. The patient presents with pain, change in vision, loss of transparency.

Very serious etiologies of keratitis are:
- Interstitial keratitis - seen with Syphilis.
- Central corneal ulcer - some very aggressive types are from fungal or pneumonia infections.
- Dendritic ulcer - caused by the Herpes Simplex virus.

The treatment is antibacterial, anti-fungal and or antiviral topical drops depending of the etiology. In some cases, steroids may be used to prevent scarring.

Corneal dystrophies are inherited conditions which are characterized a build-up of abnormal material in the cornea. Over time the cornea becomes translucent or opaque in more serious corneal dystrophies.

Corneal degeneration's - involves deterioration of the corneal tissue. Can be unilateral or bilateral. Compared to corneal dystrophies, they are not inherited. They are usually progressive and involve underlying ocular disease. During eye examination, patients present with a change in corneal shape and/or transparency that or may not affect vision. Examples of corneal degenerations include:
- **Arcus senilus** - deposit of fatty material in the limbus of the cornea, it appears like a smokey gray ring around the edge of the cornea. There is no loss of vision because it is not in the optical center of the eye. This is a common, benign condition in the elderly. However, this corneal degeneration seen in a child may indicate very high cholesterol and warrants medical investigation.
- **Keratoconus** – the central corneal fibers are weakened. Over time the pressure of the eye causes the thinned cornea to become more "cone" shaped. Females are more affected than males. The progression is variable. It may be hereditary; The person is usually diagnosed in their 2nd decade of life. In the earlier years there are frequent prescription lens changes. A more rigid contact lens is fitted when the optics of the cornea becomes more severe. The tear film helps to fill in the irregular cornea. Over time, corneal scaring may occur. In some cases, the corneal may lead to perforation or rupture. Corneal transplants may be needed in some individuals. The most common reason for a corneal transplant is Keratoconus. The prognosis for a successful corneal transplant is good.

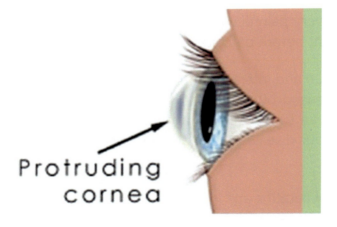

Protruding
cornea

Munson's sign – when a person with advanced Keratoconus looks down their lower eyelid protrudes out.

Band keratopathy - there is a lying down of calcium salts in the central palpebral area that causes a loss of transparency. This process is related to a lack of vitamin C. This is one of the leading causes of blindness in the world (not seen often in developed countries)

Band keratopathy image.

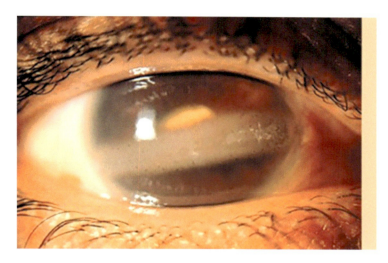

Sclera

The sclera is the tough white fibrous outer envelope of tissue covering the entire eyeball except for the cornea. Also called sclerotic, sclerotic coat.

- **Episcleritis -** is an inflammation of the top layer of the sclera, it may have an autoimmune component. Clients diagnosed with this condition are generally presented with a unilateral redness of one segment of the episclera. There may be tearing and irritation (see the redness/injection in photo below). Most of the time it only affects one eye. The etiology is usually unknown or idiopathic.

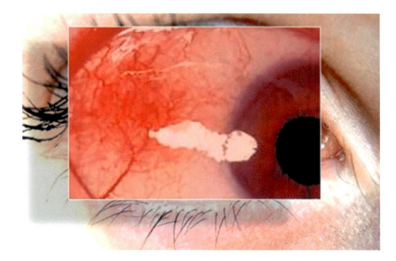

Episcleritis image (shown above, area of pink inflamed vessels in the left part of the sclera).

The treatment is anti-inflammatory drops

Scleritis – Inflammation of the sclera. **It** causes local pain and can cause vision loss. **Scleritis** can occur with diseases such as rheumatoid arthritis, Wegener's granulomatosis, gout and lupus etc.

The client presents with a painful, very injected (deep, reddish purple). The treatment is first deal with the underlying condition plus use anti-inflammatory drops. They tend to have some type of collagen disorder. In order to treat the symptoms in the sclera, the underlying condition must be treated.

Uvea Tract (little "grape")
The Uveal Tract contains 3 main structures: Iris, Ciliary body and the Choroid. During the embryogenic phase of development, these structures are developed together and have one layer of continuous tissue in common.

Anterior Uveitis - is unilateral inflammation of the iris and ciliary body. It may be caused by trauma, accompany a systemic disease (arthritis) or be idiopathic. The patient presents with:
- An acute or chronic onset of symptoms
- Miotic (small) pupil
- Differing levels of injection (redness) or ciliary flush
- Much tearing and photophobia (light sensitivity)
- Debris in the aqueous chamber (known as "cells and flare")
- Tonometry readings show the eye to be sick and soft with IOP under 12 mmHg

The treatment is to dilate the pupil, putting the iris at rest and keeps it from sticking to the lens. An anti-inflammatory (steroid) drop is also needed.

Iris Malformations are any abnormalities to the iris due to trauma or congenital formation

Albinism – no pigment in the iris. The patient presents with a pink iris and complains of photophobia (sensitivity to light/glare). Light control is important because the lack of pigment in the iris renders its ability to control illumination to the eye useless. Persons with complete or ocular albinism lack pigment in retina.

Iridodialysis/Angle Recession - trauma to the iris causing it to tear and/bleed into the anterior chamber. The red blood cells clog the trabecular meshwork, causing a secondary glaucoma.

Treatment includes topical drops and/or surgery to create an artificial drainage system may be needed for the glaucoma.

ANTERIOR CHAMBER
Glaucoma: Characterized by higher intra-ocular pressure, optic nerve head damage and resultant visual field defects. Elevated intraocular pressure - 24 mmHg or higher, usually 30 or higher. Optic nerve head damage - examination of the ONH reveals increased cupping of the disk (greater than .5 C/D).

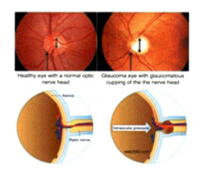

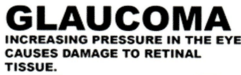

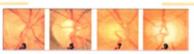

Visual field defects – the vision loss can be plotted with a visual field test. It begins with an enlarged blind spot and progresses outward, resulting in loss or peripheral vision (called tunnel vision). This loss of side vision occurs of many years (10 – 15) if left untreated.

Glaucoma is a common eye condition in which the fluid pressure inside the eye rises because of slowed fluid drainage from the Schlemm's canal

There are many types of glaucoma; they differ in signs, symptoms and presentation:

1. **Chronic open-angle glaucoma (COAG):** also called primary open angle glaucoma. COAG accounts for 85 – 90% of all the glaucoma's and is the third cause of vision impairment in the US. The angle of the eye is normal. There is probably a problem with the trabecular meshwork and the outflow of aqueous is diminished and/or too much aqueous is being produced by the ciliary processed (of the ciliary body). This is a slow, gradual (chronic) painless disease, which reduced vision over time (10 - 20 years). The visual fields are severely restricted, ultimately the central vision is destroyed and blindness results if not treated.

The treatment of glaucoma is to reduce the pressure. The symptoms are treated, it is not cured. Initial treatment is topical drops; some additional systemic medications may be also used. If medications cannot be tolerated or don't work, a procedure may be performed to improve the drainage of the aqueous (laser trabeculotomy). Other procedures used in very resistant cases are filtration surgery and cryoablation surgery.

2. **Acute angle closure glaucoma**: Researches show that acute angle closure glaucoma accounts for 10 – 15% of all the glaucoma's. With time all angles narrow due to continued growth of the lens. Pressures may rise slowly to an abnormal range over the years. Over time synechia tend to form between the iris and cornea, slowly sealing off the angle. Left untreated, an acute angle closure attack occurs resulting in very high pressures (40 – 60 mmHg). Angle closure glaucoma has a rapid onset, acute loss of corneal transparency and optic nerve injury. The pain is quite extreme, the patient may be vomiting and have extreme headaches. This is an ocular emergency. The visual acuity loss may be severe.

Patient with narrow angles glaucoma and raised IOP (before an acute angle closure attack), can have a laser procedure to reduce the production of aqueous by the ciliary body or to increase the drainage. Topical drops are used to keep the pressures below normal.

3. **Secondary open-angle glaucoma**: This glaucoma is secondary to another eye disease such as rubeosis iridis, eye trauma.
4. **Congenital glaucoma** - the child is born with a malformed angle.
5. **Normal Tensive Glaucoma** – also called normal or low-pressure glaucoma. The patient has a normal angle and IOP in the normal range (10 – 22mmhg). Patients with low-pressure glaucoma experience optic nerve damage and progressive visual field losses. These individuals may have pre-existing systemic conditions (such as diabetes), which reduce the perfusion (supply of nutrients) to the optic nerve.

Other Internal Conditions in The Eye

Before you consider pathological images, below is a photo of a normal fundus (back of the eye).

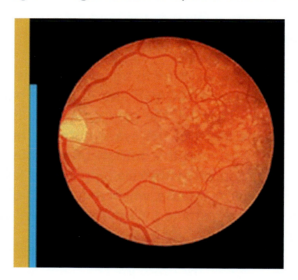

The blood vessels look like rivers flowing and branching out. The optic nerve head is **a yellowish pink**, sharply demarcated by the reddish retina. The macular area is **a darker red**, with the darkest area in the center being the foveola. There is black pigment indicating scarring, no blurring, and no red hemorrhaging. The fundus is clearly viewed.

RETINOPATHY OF PREMATURITY (ROP) FORMERLY CALLED RETROLENTAL FIBROPLASIA (RLF)

This is the leading cause of blindness in children in the United States (US). It is typically seen among premature infants (Development of the retinal blood vessel system (vasculature) is not complete until the 9th month of gestation). It is sometimes found in full term infants – risk factors include blood transfusions, acidosis, septicemia and intraventricular hemorrhage.

These children receive too much oxygen which can lead to the followings:

- Constriction of retinal blood vessels
- Severe spasm and damage to retinal blood vessels
- Secondary proliferation of vessels and glial tissue

In advanced stages, the pupil of the eye will appear white. This is because the area behind the pupil is filled with a retinal tissue mass from the detached retina.

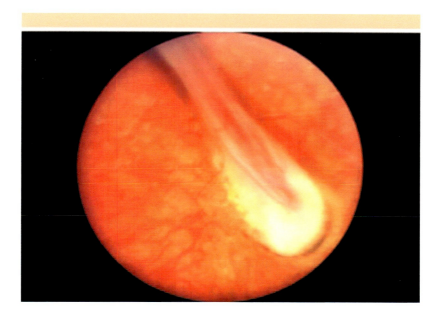

In the above photo, there is a proliferation of tissue in the bottom right corner. It is pulling on the retina – This is stage 3 of ROP.

ROP Stages
Stage 1: (minor changes) There are retinal changes at a demarcation line between the vascularized and the avascularized retina

Stage 2: (disc distortion) A very distinct ridge of tissue is formed

Stage 3: (retinal fold) There is a proliferation of opaque tissue and retinal vessels

Stage 4: (incomplete retrolental mass) Proliferation is severe, retina becomes detached

Stage 5: (complete retrolental mass) - Total retinal detachment.

ROP can spontaneously resolve even up to stage 3. Retinal Cryotherapy or photocoagulation is initiated at stage 3 plus to save vision. If patients retain vision, they tend to have high amounts of myopia. Secondary problems include glaucoma (the mass of tissue blocks the proper flow of the aqueous out of the eye).

RETINAL DETACHMENT (RD)

In this situation, a portion of the retina detaches from its supporting structure (neural form non-neural retina or retina from the choroid (at Bruch's membrane). The most serious detachment is superior because gravity works against the patient accelerating the detachment. Generally, RD is due to injuries from trauma, diabetic retinopathy and degenerative retinal conditions. This is another **true ocular emergency**. The retina can only be separated from its nutritional source a matter of hours to days (depending on location).

Signs and symptoms:
- Flashing lights followed by spots (floaters)
- Sometimes the patient reports pain
- Poor night vision
- Decreased visual acuity (if the macula is affected)
- Mobility and travel problems (from lateral retinal detachment)
- Retina appears fuzzy
- Edema of the retina

While the physical reattachment surgery is very successful, this does not mean the patient will have a good vision. Visual prognosis is related to time away from the retina's source of nutrition. The macula, the highest consumer of oxygen is at most risk; the side retina is of a lesser risk.

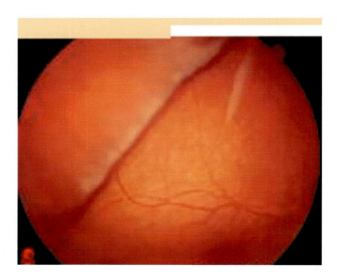

MACULAR HOLE

This is a hole in macular/foveal area. There is a tear or opening in the macula. As the hole forms, things in your central vision will look blurry, wavy or distorted. As the hole grows, a dark or blind spot appears in your central vision. A macular hole does not affect your peripheral (side) vision. It may happen spontaneously in older patients. Generally, its dues to prolonged edema in the macular area or traction by a membrane.

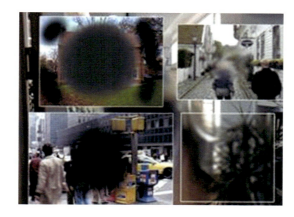

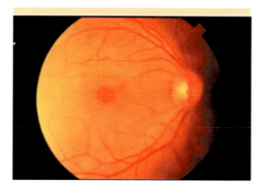

Above, the outline of a hole appears in the center of the macula area – this is the macular hole

Signs and symptoms:
- Loss of vision directly proportional to the size of the hole
- Gradual decline in the central (straight-ahead) vision of affected eye. Straight lines or objects look bent or wavy.
- Difficulty with reading and other near tasks.

RETINITIS PIGMENTOSA (RP)

Retinitis pigmentosa (RP) is an inherited disorder that results from harmful changes in any one of more than 50 genes. These genes carry the instructions for making proteins that are needed in cells within the retina, called photoreceptors. Some of the changes, or mutations, within genes are so severe that the gene cannot make the required protein, limiting the cell's function. Other mutations produce a protein that is toxic to the cell. Still other mutations lead to an abnormal protein that doesn't function properly. In all three cases, the result is damage to the photoreceptors. There are many forms of RP, which makes the prognosis for ultimate visual acuity difficult to predict.

With RP, something is happening at the site of the outer segments of the rods. The used outer discs start to accumulate around the outer segments preventing nutrition to the rod. Photoreceptor death occurs. Pigment migrates to areas of cell death. In RP there is much destruction of the rods, which is indicated by the extensive pigmentary clumping (depicted in the image below).

Symptoms
Retinitis pigmentosa usually starts in childhood. But exactly when it starts and how quickly it gets worse varies from person to person. It's is noticeable in 3rd decade with a progression to severe vision loss by the 5th decade. Most people with RP lose much of their sight by early adulthood. Then by age 40, they are often legally blind.

When vision loss occurs in childhood, the retinal degeneration often leads to total blindness. RP is seen with many congenital syndromes (i.e., Usher's syndrome, Lawrence-Moon-Bidel syndrome). The presence of RP can be detected early with electrodiagnostic testing (the signal is reduced during electroretinogram (ERG) testing). Genetic counseling is important for those considering having children.

The dark black clumps of pigment indicate the atrophy/death of the rods. This is referred to as bone spicules (or bear tracking).

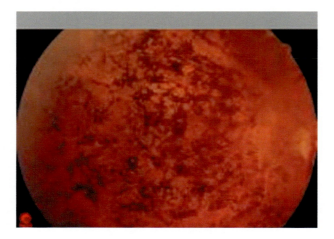

MACULAR DEGENERATION
Macular degeneration is a progressive vision impairment resulting from deterioration of the central part of retina, known as macula. Most people with macular degeneration have the more common type, dry AMD, in one or both eyes. In one out of ten people, dry AMD progresses to wet AMD. There is also juvenile form (JMD) which can be categorized as Stargardts Disease and Best's Disease. These are congenital diseases, which are expressed in youth.

1. **Stargardts Diseases**

This form of JMD is bilaterally symmetrical in nature and has a progressive loss of central vision. The macula involved first, usually between ages 6 and 20. The degeneration can extend into the peripheral retina. The macula has beaten or scrambled egg appearance. The early form of Stargardts disease is known as fundus flavimaculatus, which looks like yellow fishtails in the macula. The visual acuity is typically 20/200. If the involvement extends beyond the macula, the VA will be greater than 20/200.

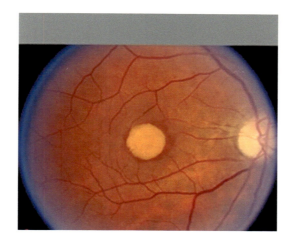

There is a disturbance (yellowish in nature like a scrambled egg) in the macular area and a little beyond.

2. **Vitelliform Macular Degeneration (Best's disease)** It is also hereditary with an onset between 5 and 15 years of age. The macula is described as having an egg yolk lesion (like a sunny side up egg). Later on in the disease hemorrhages and scarring is seen in the macula. This vision loss is less severe with Best's disease. The VA is rarely worse than 20/200.

AGE-RELATED MACULOPATHY (ARM)

There are essentially two forms of AMD. It used to be described as the dry and wet forms of AMD. Today, we describe ARM in terms as non-exudative and exudative types. Exudates are from fluids that leak out of blood vessels.

In the Non-Exudative (Dry Type):
- The client/patient experiences a bilateral (both eyes) loss of vision.
- It usually affects persons 70 years of age and older.
- The fundus looks mottled in the macula area. The pigmented epithelium becomes disorganized.
- There is drusen (hard whitish/yellow deposit) just under or around the macula
- There is NO bleeding or hemorrhaging. The drusen mostly likely prevents the macula from its nutrition and the macular cells die.
- This type of ARM comprises 90% of all ARM.

In the Exudative (Wet Type):
- The resultant loss of central vision is faster.
- Choroidal vessels leak exudates (fluid and or blood) under, in and around the macular. This creates a hypoxic condition, which leads to vessel proliferation in the macula. Hemorrhage and or detachment result from the new macular vessels.
- The vision loss may be mild or severe.
- If detected early enough, ophthalmic surgeons seal the leaking vessels with laser treatment. Anothernewer treatment is photodynamic therapy. A light sensitive medicine

(verteporfin) is injected into a patient's arm and it goes to the body to the eyes. Then a non-thermal laser is shined into the eyes. The verteporfin causes a chemical reaction, which destroys the leaking, abnormal blood vessels. This type of photodynamic therapy can help manage blood leaking from choroidal vessels through the RPE.
- There is a resultant macular scar and permanent loss of vision

The exudative type accounts for about 10% of all ARM. It often affects people who are younger, 50 years of age and older. Some of the non-exudative ARM can develop exudative ARM though this is less likely.

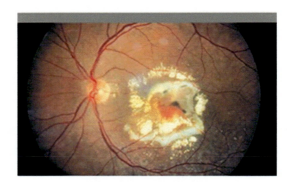

SYSTEMIC DISEASES WITH OCULAR COMPLICATIONS
1. **AIDS (Acquired Immune Deficiency Syndrome:**

The HIV (human immunodeficiency virus) virus causes AIDS. Ocular complications occur in 75% of individuals with AIDS.

The four main types of ocular problems include:
- CMV (cytomegalovirus) retinitis
- Keratitis
- Herpes Zoster
- Herpes Simplex

2. **Hypertension (high blood pressure:**

Typically, the etiology of hypertension is unknown. Stress can have a negative or compounding effect on high blood pressure. Sustained high blood pressure causes sclerosis of the arteries and arterioles in the body, including the eye.

These hypertensive changes are reversible. Over time, the arteriole walls become hardened or sclerosed. These sclerotic changes are irreversible.

In early stages of hypertensive retinopathy (HR), there is a narrowing of the arterioles. The sections of the veins experience a very localized constriction that can pull on and deviate the normal direction of the vein. At this point there may be hemorrhage and fluid leakage (exudates). In advanced stages there is edema around the optic nerve head (papilledema) and in and around the macular causing a macular star.

3. **Arteriolar Sclerosis (AS):**

Sustained hypertension causes irreversible changes in the arterioles known as Arteriolar Sclerosis.

The changes are in the arteriole walls. At first there is a change in the reflection of light. The normal reflex seen when looking inside the eye is widened. The arteriole walls are being hardening and they are heavier. Remember arteries always cross veins (they are on top of the veins). As the arterioles become heavier and heavier, they start to press on the veins. The arterioles normally red in color (because they are transparent) start to look coppery colored. The arteries start to compress the veins, veins may become nicked. In advanced stages, the arteries are opaque and so look like silver wires. There is marked compression on the veins (cause A-V compression).

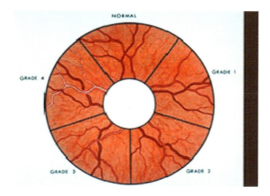

4. **Congenital Rubella:**

Usually the infected mother transmits the benign rubella (German measles) virus to the fetus. The earlier in the pregnancy this occurs, the more serious the complications and malformations.

Ocular problems associated with congenital Rubella are:
- Retinopathy – salt and pepper fundus
- Cataract
- Microphthalmos
- Glaucoma
- Nystagmus
- Less common ocular conditions are iritis, corneal clouding, iritis and extreme refractive errors.

5. **Degenerative Myopia**

This inherited condition causes extreme nearsightedness (more than 20 Diopters). It is also called pathological or malignant myopia. The normal eye is pretty much adult size during early childhood. Refractive errors such as hyperopia or myopia are stable by early adulthood. However, the sclera of a person with degenerative myopia continues to grow posteriorly. The eye lengthens which stretches the posterior pole of the eye. This abnormally stretches the retina and choroid over time. Degeneration of the retina may occur early or late in life.

This condition leads the following signs and symptoms:
- Patients experience frequent changes (increases) in prescriptions due to the ever-increasing myopia
- Retinal tears occurred as the retina is stretched more and more
- Persons with degenerative myopia are at greater risk for retinal detachments
- There is a corresponding visual field loss to the area of degeneration or retinal detachment
- Degenerative myopia is hereditary

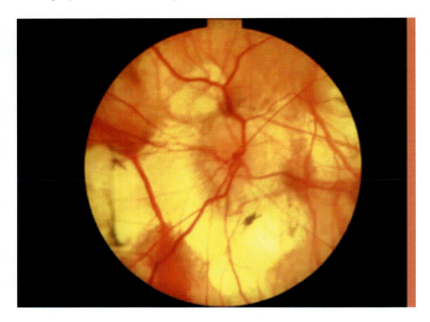

6. **Central Retinal Artery (CRA) Occlusion:**

Central retinal artery (CRA) occlusion is a disease of the eye where the flow of blood through the central retinal artery is blocked (occluded). There are several different causes of this occlusion; the most common is carotid artery atherosclerosis.

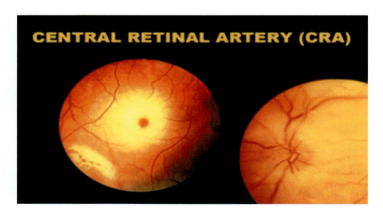

This is another true ocular emergency. Time is of the essence. Oxygen must be re-established to the retina. If the entire retinal artery is occluded, there will be a sudden loss of vision. If a CRA branch is blocked, the vision loss may go unnoticed (especially if is in the side retina).

Signs and Symptoms:
- Sudden blindness in one or both eyes.
- Sudden blurring of vision in one or both eyes.
- Gradual loss of vision.

Since, the central retinal artery brings blood, oxygen and nutrients to the eye. It provides nutrition to the outer 2/3 of the retina. If the CRA occluded, no blood is getting into the eye. The retina will therefore be very pale. The arteries will look threadlike (little to no blood in them). The veins will also be very fragmented. There is a bright red spot, the macula that stands out in the pale retina. The macula is red because its blood supply is from the Choriocapillaris (which arise from the choroidal vessels).

7. **Central Retinal Vein Occlusion**
When the main retinal vein becomes blocked, it is called central retinal vein occlusion (CRVO).

When the vein is blocked, blood and fluid spill out into the retina. The macula can swell from this fluid, affecting your central vision. Eventually, without blood circulation, nerve cells in the eye can die and you can lose more vision.

This is another ocular emergency. Because the central retinal vein drains the blood from each of the eyes, if it is blocked, blood cannot get out from the eye. Since the blood is still coming into the eye from the CRA, there is an enormous amount of blood that backs up into the eye. This causes what is called a "bucket of blood" appearance.

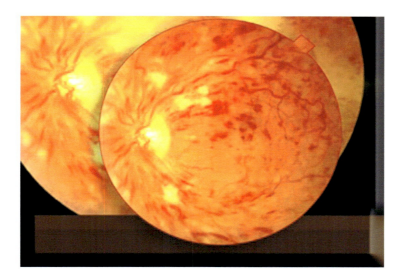

In the photo above, it is not surprising to see the veins looking engorged, edema in the eye, hemorrhaging in the retina (at the nerve fiber layer)

Signs and Symptoms:
- Vision loss or blurry vision in part or all of one eye. It can happen suddenly or become worse over several hours or days. Sometimes, you can lose all vision suddenly.

- Floaters. These are dark spots, lines or squiggles in your vision. These are shadows from tiny clumps of blood leaking into the vitreous from retinal vessels.
- Engorgement (filling of) veins
- Fluid/edema
- Large hemorrhages in nerve fiber layer of the retina
- Rupture of large vessel causing the bucket of blood appearance
- Hemorrhage must break through into the vitreous - vitreal hemorrhage

The CVRO is usually due to thrombosis (most common) or it associated with arteriosclerosis of CRA.

8. **Diabetes Mellitus**

#1 cause of visual impairments:
- Metabolic disorder
- Juvenile - congenital deficiency of Beta cells
- Senile - hyaline degeneration
- Slight preference for females (obese, over 40, non-white) Inherited
- Third leading cause of death

Ocular Changes:
- Xanthelasmas - fatty plaques in skin of eyelids
- Ptosis
- Paralysis of extraocular muscles
- III nerve palsy
- Rubeosis irides
- Diabetic cataract
- Asteroid hyalosis
- Diabetic retinopathy
- Optic atrophy

Diabetic Retinopathy (DR)
- Complication in long-standing diabetes (unless there is optimal blood sugar control)
- 95 % of diabetics (10-15 years) develop some form of DR
- After 20 years, nearly all patients with type 1 and 60% with type 2 have some degree of retinopathy.
- 2 phases: Non-proliferative Retinopathy and Proliferative phases with different stages based on the severity of the condition. See image below:

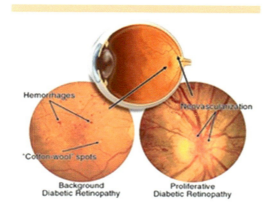

- Central vision may be impaired by macular edema or capillary nonperfusion
- New blood vessels from DR and pulling of fibrous tissue and lead to a retinal detachment (tract.)
- Leakage of blood from new blood vessels

Diabetics have a 90% chance of retaining vision when the retina is treated before severe damage.

Fluorescein angiography may be ordered with macular edema. Special dye is injected into the arm. Pictures are taken of the eye as the fluid passes through the vasculature, leaking vessels are detected. Timely laser surgery can reduce vision loss from macular edema by 50%. A focal laser treatment is aimed directly onto the damaged blood vessel to seal it and prevent it from leaking. This will need to be done more than once.

A vitrectomy is performed for vitreal hemorrhage. The vitreous is replaced by saline or an oily substance

Excellent glucose control can reduce or eliminate the risk of developing retinopathy and nephropathy.

9. **Syphilis**

Syphilis is an infection caused by the bacterium Treponema pallidum subspecies pallidum. Adults with acquired syphilis can have severe vision problems due to inflammation and infection of the choroid (choroiditis). The clinical picture is often referred to as a "salt and pepper" fundus. The salt refers to seeing the sclera and the pepper refers to seeing accumulated pigment (which migrates to areas of destruction). The areas missing are healthy retina and choroid – which explains the vision loss.

Children born with hereditary syphilis (from infected mothers) get a severe keratitis called Interstitial Keratitis. The age of onset is around 10-13 years old.

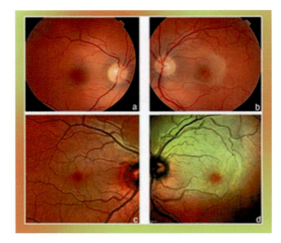

Image of Syphilis.
In the image above, there is scarring (black pigment clumping) from the damage to the retina from the syphilis. The pigment as always denotes scarring from the damaged area.

10. **Toxoplasmosis**

Toxoplasmosis is a parasitic disease caused by Toxoplasma gondii. The source is typically an infected rodent (mouse) though the cat is usually blamed. Poultry (chickens) are also a common source. Generally, a person is infected when getting scratched by the infected cat. The Toxoplasmosis can be transmitted via inhalation, ingestion or blood...

Toxoplasmosis has a predilection for **macular tissue**. Commonly there is a rather large lesion of the macular area, which results in a huge macular scar. If looks like someone "punched" out the macular area. Other parts of the retina can be affected, though a large macula lesion is more typical.

Hereditary toxoplasmosis is much more involved. Toxoplasmosis likes neural and macular tissue. There is often a central nervous systems (CNS) involvement. Macula lesions with here become evident at 10-15 years of age. There may also be a choroiditis. Vision loss is related to areas affected.

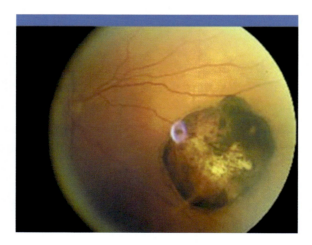

In the photo above there is a huge "punched out" macular scar typical to Toxoplasmosis. In this case, the patient would have a big macular/perimacular scotoma.

11. **Histoplasmosis**

Histoplasmosis is an infection caused by breathing in spores of a fungus often found in bird and bat droppings. This fungus grows best in certain temperature zones around the world (often found in the Mississippi Valley area, South America). In the eye, it results in an inflammation of the retina. Clinically the retina has many small-infected areas called histospots. The most common culprit is from the feces of chickens. It is uniocular but can become binocular

There may be a central lesion or lesions in or around the macula. There is an area of hemorrhage around the lesion – this is the histospot. Unfortunately, this fungus affects around optic nerve head in 70-85% of the cases. This would result in very poor vision. Remember that the axons from the entire retina area collected and leave the eye via the optic nerve. We also see multiple histospots in the peripheral retina.

In this photo, there are healed histoplasmosis spots.

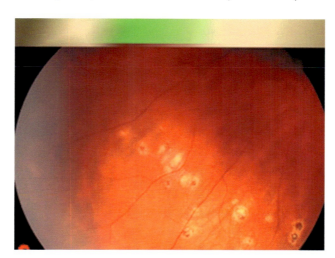

12. **Toxocariasis**

According to CDC (Centers for Disease Control and prevention), Toxocariasis is an infection transmitted from animals to humans (zoonosis) caused by the parasitic roundworms commonly found in the intestine of dogs (Toxocara canis) and cats (T. cati).

This disease affects children who eat mud pies (so called dirt eaters). Once ingested, the worm eggs hatch in intestine and travel throughout the body. In the eye, the worm ends up in the retina. It becomes quite large. The eye has a reaction to the decaying carcass and retinal destruction is a result of the inflammatory process. It affects 4-16-year old. Toxocariasis usually affects only one eye in 70% of cases.

13. **Cortical Visual Impairment (CVI)**

Generally, cortical visual impairment (CVI) refers to a decreased visual response due to a neurological problem affecting the visual part of the Brain. Typically, an individual with CVI has a normal eye exam or has an eye condition that cannot account for the abnormal visual behavior. In this way, the nature of the disruption of vision caused by this damage correlates to location and extent of the injury itself. This explains why the visual abilities and disabilities of individuals with CVI vary greatly.

How a CVRT/LVT/O&M may prepare his/her environment to assess an individual with CVI? What materials will be needed to adapt?

In order to assess and provide interventions for individuals with CVI, we must first be familiar with the following: **strong color preference** (especially for red or yellow), **need for movement** to elicit or sustain visual attention, **visual latency, visual field preferences** (the presence of unusual field locations in addition to loss of visual field), **difficulties with visual complexity, light-gazing and non-purposeful gaze, difficulty with distance viewing, absent or atypical visual reflexes, difficulty with visual novelty** and **absence of visually guided reach** (the ability to look at and touch an object at the same time is not displayed, and these two actions are performed separately). In general, the greater the severity of CVI, the greater the number of CVI characteristics present. However, these characteristics may change or improve. It is important to make sure that the environment supports the individual's ability to pay attention to visual stimuli.

A CVRT/LVT can prepare the environment according to the three phases of CVI progression:
Possible Environmental Considerations at Level I
- Precaution about "Vision Stimulation"
- For the individual who is in Phase I of building resolution, he/she would visually attend:
  - to familiar objects (usually one color)
  - when there are no sound distracters
  - when there are no visual distracters
  - other sensory inputs are carefully controlled
  - when room light is low

In the same way, in order to use vision in a more stable or consistent way, significant support from the environment will be required. For environment with difficulty to control (client home, student classroom, or a clinical facility), we may use occluders, sunglasses (NoIR or Cocoones Lenses} and shiny/reflective and/or moving objects.

Possible Environmental Considerations at Level II
- For the individual who is in Phase II of building resolution, he/she can attend:
  - to objects that share features of color or pattern with the "familiar" objects
  - when familiar or low intensity auditory inputs compete
  - on increased pattern/object beyond 3-4 feet
  - to different lighting situations (not overly attentive to lights)

In Level II environments, near surfaces must still remain free of visual clutter. Based on the individual's level of visual functioning, materials from phase I can also be used for this phase.

Possible Environmental Considerations at Level III: In addition to Level II, heighten contrast and reduction of complexity

Overall, **a CVRT/LVT should develop environmental checklists** that raise awareness of certain aspects of the environment that may need to be modified for specific individuals:
- Is the environment familiar?
- Is the room safe (uncluttered pathways, safe corners/edges...etc.
- Lighting conditions (lighting consideration are not only important as related to visual conditions but also to states of arousal, both of concern for clients with CVI or TBI)
- Auditory conditions (TV, radio, phone ringing, traffic noise, people talking, overall impressions of noise conditions...etc.)
- Room Temperature (hot, cool, or cold) ....

Two intervention tasks/activities that can be used to improve visual functioning:

1- Phase III – This phase refers to good use of vision for most tasks but may have difficulty with complex environment and with distance viewing. Individuals in this phase (score from about 7 1/2 to 10 on the CVI range) use vision in performing most tasks. This is the resolution of all CVI characteristics.

A 12-year-old girl diagnosed with CVI secondary to anoxia from surgery during infancy. When at school or at her local library she may need to use a card with a cut-out window to isolate target images or she may need to use a highlighter with a marker to draw attention to them. In this situation, she can also use occludes or window cards to block out excess detail on a page of image or symbols. With the marker, she can highlight critical picture by using color that could help improve her visual functioning ability.

2 – Phase II – This phase refers to the integration visions with functions (score from 4 to 7 on the CVI range).

A 6-year-old boy diagnosed with CVI who requires an environment in which objects share features of color. In this case, during lunch at school, the 6-year-old boy can position to sort yellow and red spoons placed against a black background and can do so while other student activities are occurring within the classroom.

14. **Hemianopsia**
This is caused by stroke or some mechanical or vascular obstruction, which presses on the optic nerve pathways after the eye on the way to the visual cortex of the brain. With this condition there is half field of vision in both eyes (right, left, upper or lower). The field of vision is divided right down the midline of vision. The reason for such a pattern is that retinal fibers cross after each optic nerve leaves the eye on its way to the visual area of the brain.

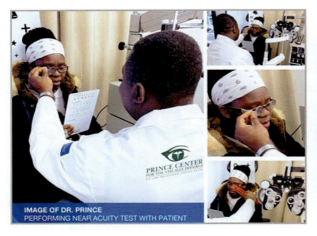

IMAGE OF DR. PRINCE
PERFORMING NEAR ACUITY TEST WITH PATIENT

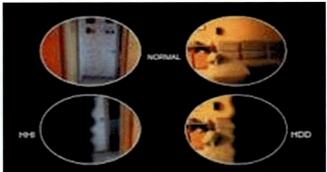

Common functional problems:
- Loss of half of visual field
- Reading difficulties
- Right hemianopsia - the person is reading into their scotoma
- Left hemianopsia - the person may lose their place, they may miss the left side of the page and insteadstart reading from the middle of the page to the end and back again)

Management Strategies:
- Fresnel prisms
- Read using the thumb, paper clips or a bold straight line as a marker for the beginning or end of a line(right hemianopsia)
- Read in upside down or vertical fusion (minimizes the blind field in right hemianopsia)

Secondary Optic Atrophy

Secondary optic atrophy is degeneration of optic nerve secondary to retinal disease, i.e.: glaucoma, CRA occlusion, CRV occlusion, Retinitis Pigmentosa, diabetic retinopathy). The optic nerve degeneration is a complication of the retinal disease.

Signs and symptoms:
- Loss of vision itself
- The optic nerve head is pale; this disc pallor is related to the extent of the atrophy (cell death)
- With optic atrophy, the changes in visual functioning happen very slowly over time which makes it difficult for the eye care specialist to predict the progression of the atrophy and the final visual prognosis.

Leber's Optic Atrophy

Rare

- Inherited (maternal DNA mutation)
- Rare condition
- Optic neuropathy more common in 20-30-year-old males
- Present unilaterally, becomes bilateral within months
- Some vision retained, vision impairment is varying
- Central scotoma is common

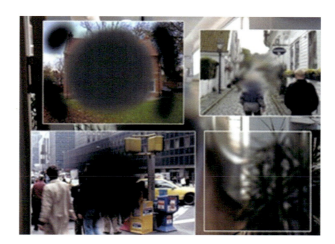

Chapter 4:
Normal changes in the Aging Eye and Functional Implications

Just as our physical strength decreases with age, our eyes also exhibit age-related decline in performance, particularly as we reach our 60's and beyond. In other words, as we get older, our eyes and vision change over time. There is a normal age-related change in anatomy and physiology of the structure of the eye. *The number of endothelial cells that keep the cornea at the correct concentration of water (78% and hence, transparent) is decreased by 67% by 80 years of age.* This will lead to loss of corneal sensitivity. The situation is not different with the other structures of the eye which also change as we get older:

- **Pupil and Iris**: Pupils become mitotic (very small) due to weakness of the dilator muscle and sclerosis of the stroma of the iris. This limits the amount of light entering the eye.
- **The crystalline lens** loses its elasticity and flexibility beginning in the 40's. This loss will lead to a decrease of the ability to see objects clearly at near.
- Jelly-like substance of **the vitreous** starts to liquefy and shrink as we get older (50's and 60's). This explains the presence of a greater number of floaters or spots.
- **The Retina**: The blood vessel supplying the retina loses their elasticity and become atherosclerotic which lead to a reduction of light absorbing pigment and visual acuity. These changes can lead to a number of noticeable differences in how well we see. However, the age-related vision changes vary from one individual to another one.

The common vision problems that impact older adults are as follows:
- Presbyopia: As we get older (40+), many of us may notice difficulty in focusing on objects up close due to hardening of the lens inside the eye.
- Floaters, Dry eyes and tearing are all vision problems that can impact older adults during their daily living activity and needs immediate attention from an eye care specialist to avoid any other complication of the structure of the eye.
- Cataract: Even though cataracts are considering an age-related eye disease, they are so common among seniors that they can also be classified as a normal eye change. It's considered as the cloudy areas that cover part or the entire lens.
- Macular degeneration or age-related macular degeneration is the leading cause of blindness among American seniors.
- Other conditions include glaucoma, and diabetic retinopathy, corneal disease and eyelid problems etc.

How could these problems impact the activities of daily living?
Anyone of the above eye conditions related to age would impact older adults' daily living activities. These eye conditions could interfere with the individual's safety and ability to understand his/her surrounding during daily activities and impact the overall comfort and freedom (independence) of the individual. An individual diagnosed with cataract or diabetic retinopathy might have difficulties to perform personal and home management activities like grooming/makeup, take blood pressure and medication, money identification, telling time, telephone use, food preparation and cleaning etc. For example, with cataract, the light might not be able to get through lens as easily and, as a result, vision can be impaired. In this way, the individual might experience blurry vision and not be able to read small print at near without aid. The presence of glare could be a big issue for the individual. In situation of glaucoma, the optic nerve can be damage and lead to permanent vision loss and blindness if not taking care of properly.

Overall the individual might experience issues with the following:
- **Accommodation:** *inability to focus and see objects a near distance*
- **Sensitivity to light**: older adults will need greater amount of light than young individual when making a phone call
- **Dark adaptation**: older adults will take longer to do makeup when coming from daylight environment into a darker one
- **Color sensitivity**: an older individual might have difficulty to identify clothing in his/ her closet when going to a function.

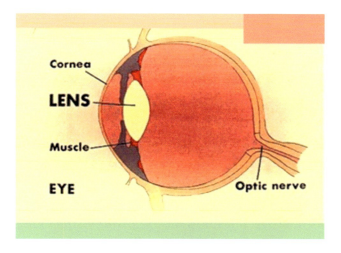

Chapter 5:
Traumatic Brain Injury (TBI) and Comprehensive Vision Rehabilitation Evaluation

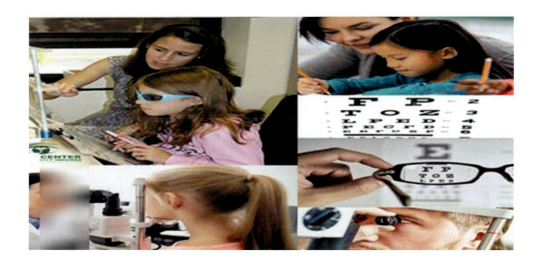

Current research indicates that a great percentage of patients diagnosed with TBI (traumatic brain injury) are struggling with vision deficits which are a direct result of their injury. Depending on its location and severity TBI can affect your vision by damaging parts of the brain involved in visual processing and/or perception (e.g., cranial nerves, optic nerve tract or other circuitry involved in vision, occipital lobe) Generally, Vision Rehabilitation Professionals Therapists may be the first to notice the problem. A functional low vision examination will accurately measure how the patient's vision works in the real world - how it functions in day-to-day living. It's not only about how well he/she can see an eye chart, but also how well he/she can see faces, street signs, newspaper print, stove dials and all the other visual clues that guide you through the day. The low vision exam he/she use his/her functional vision more effectively. It will help determine whether special low vision optical devices, better lighting, large print reading materials or other types of training through vision rehabilitation services that can help with his/her visual impairment.

Another important aspect of the low vision examination is that it gives the vision professional team the information needed in order to help the clients/patients adapt emotionally to their vision loss. For example, optimal refractive correction can make a big difference in the final corrected visual acuity and visual functioning. In addition to all the tests performed by Eye Care Specialists specializing in vision rehabilitation for TBI Client/patient, visual focusing skills along with binocular and depth perception must have special considerations in cases related to strokes, motor vehicle accidents, concussions/whiplash injuries, status-post neurosurgery for tumor resection or aneurism repairs. Of all the sensory deficits that can occur as a result of stroke, impairments of the tactile and visual systems appear to be the most common. Because both of these systems have a significant impact on motor performance, it is important to complete a thorough evaluation of each system. In this manual, our focus will be on the visual system which is frequently affected by neurologic loss. Much has been written over the years about the visual deficits resulting from stroke and brain injury. Impairments that may occur are visual perceptual paralysis resulting in diplopia, and visual perceptual deficits such as unilateral inattention based on the area of the brain affected. The selection of effective evaluation modifications to aid in diagnosing these deficits for the stroke patient with aphasia or apraxia is quite challenging to the eye care specialist and well worth the effort. It is particularly rewarding to both the patient and the practitioner when the patient had been previously labeled as untestable. The majority of TBI patients has some forms of visual field defects which be either absolute or relative. The location of a visual field defect is usually classified as central or peripheral depending on eccentricity: how far away from straight ahead it is. Defects beyond about 30 degrees eccentricity are considered to be midperipheral. Defects located within 30 degrees of straight ahead are considered central...etc. Additional descriptions of field defect location would include whether the defect is to the right, left, above, or below the persons line of sight. Sometimes the defect is described as located either nasally or temporally to indicate whether it is nearer to the nose or to the side of the head. The location is often further classified as unilateral or bilateral to describe whether visual fields are affected in one or both eyes. When a defect is bilateral, term homonymous may be used to indicate that the same side of the visual field is affected for each eye. When the field defect in one eye is on the opposite side of fixation as the defect or the other eye, the defects may be described as binasal or bitemporal, depending on which parts of the field are impaired. Some peripheral field defects are described as altitudinal, meaning that the defect involves either the upper (superior) or lower (inferior field). Other field losses are described as concentric, meaning that field has been lost symmetrically from all sides. Based on the severity and location of the injury in the brain, the client may present with the following:

- Difficulty with reading (or any activity required near vision),
- Inability to bring the two eyes together at near range
- Difficulty with Indoor and outdoor mobility
- *Double Vision*
- Visual Scanning or Tracking Problems
- Deficit of eye movement leading to *Nystagmus, imbalance and dizziness*

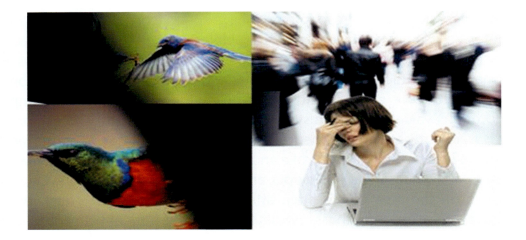

As well illustrated in the above image, the brain of this client interprets the world as if it was moving, (known as *oscillopsia*), because of this newly acquired, involuntary, oculomotor deficit.

Management consist of vision rehabilitation therapy. Reading or progressive lenses and/or prisms.

Acquired visual perceptual deficits

No image is perceived as unique or isolated. Seeing something involves assigning it place in the whole: a location in space, a score on the scale of size or brightness or distance. A basic understanding of sensory integrative functioning along with the visual perception skills are essential to a well-planned program of vision stimulation for children diagnosed with acquired visual perceptual deficits. To quote Professor Dr. Audrey Smith: *"It's the process by which the central nervous system coordinates input from sensory receptors throughout the body, associates this input with stored memories of prior experiences, and produces adaptive responses to life situations".* In other word: information is receiving (input of sensory receptors), then perceiving (organizing input into information) then interpreting (Recalling and comparing experiences to past memories) then planning (adaptive responses to life situations) and acting. (Look at Me, pg 46, 2001). In the same way, vision rehab professional must master the visual perception skills to better manage clients coming to their practice with this type of deficit. Visual perception skills include the following:

- Visual closure abilities
- Part-whole relationships
- Pattern recognition
- Figure-ground discrimination
- Spatial orientation

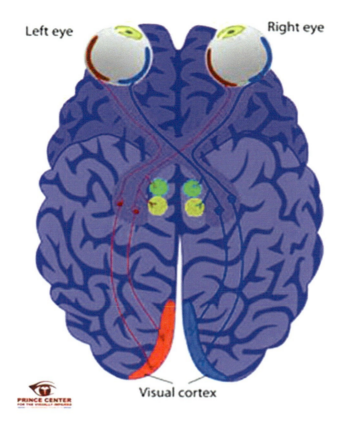

Many patients diagnosed with TBI (Traumatic Brain Injury) develop some form of deficits of the above skills, which often create visual confusion and difficulty understanding visual information. They may exhibit decreased of visual discrimination, figure-ground, visual memory, and spatial relations. Patients with visual closure deficit are often unable to identify and recognize objects or symbols with complete representation. Their reading comprehension are often affected and may even not be able to remember things they see.

In conclusion, a thorough functional visual assessment by vision rehab specialist is necessary for patients struggling with the aftermath of a traumatic head injury.

Dealing with post traumatic brain injury (Stroke) adult Clients (Patients):
A successful interaction between a client (patient) and an effective helper (Nurse, counselor or CNA) requires that the helper possess and demonstrate the following identifiable characteristics:
1. **Sensitivity**: is not taught or acquired, it is felt and experienced. It involves awareness and understanding and is exclusive of judgment.
2. **Empathy:** should not be confused with sympathy. Empathy is seeing the client's world from the client's perspective. It is the utilization of the skills of reflective listening to hear the client accurately. It involves the use of influencing skills and the sharing of oneself and expertise, only as much as the client can absorb and within the client's frame of reference.

3. **Positive regard**: is unconditional and involves selective attention to the positive aspects of the client's verbalization and behavior. It is the recognition of the client's assets.
4. **Respect:** involves making enhancing, positive statements to the client and encouraging the client to move forward. It includes honest appreciation of and toleration for differences.
5. **Warmth:** primarily is expressed nonverbally. It is the use of vocal tone, posture, and facial expression to denote that helper cares for the client.
6. **Concreteness:** means being specific, obtaining details, and requesting clarification of facts and feelings
7. **Immediacy:** is responding to the client in the same tense (present, past, or future) that the client uses.
8. **Confrontation**: is meeting the client directly and pointing out differences, mixed messages, incongruities, and discrepancies in verbal and nonverbal behavior. Confrontation should not be seen as expressing a different opinion, no matter how helpful the Nurse or Counselor thinks it may be
9. **Genuineness**: is being truly yourself in relationship with others, being spontaneous, and being ensitive to, without being engulfed by, the needs of the client.

Chapter 6:
Inside the Low Vision Exam

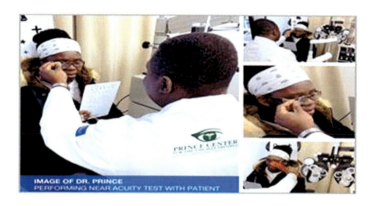

IMAGE OF DR. PRINCE
PERFORMING NEAR ACUITY TEST WITH PATIENT

What tests are performed in a low vision exam?
The tests performed in a low vision exam are:
- Case history (optional)
- Distance visual acuities
- Near visual acuities (evaluation of near vision and reading skills)
- Amber grid testing
- Color vision testing and glare sensitivity if it pertains to the patient's symptoms)
- Visual/mobility field testing
- Contrast sensitivity testing
- Refraction
- Binocular vision evaluation
- Keratometry
- Eye health evaluation
- Magnification/optical devices

Case History: Although it may not be considered as a test, the health history of the client must be conducted before any testing is performed. It consist of the chiefs compliant, last eye examination, visual/ocular history, distance visual abilities (present and past), independent travel concerns, near visual abilities (present and past), social/emotional review, general health review, environmental challenges (present and past), education and/or vocation and avocation (present and past) needs, special visual goals and desires in a prioritized order. With the information from the history, we should have a feel for the handicapping effect of the client's visual loss.

Distance Visual Acuities: This will help establish the patient's baseline ability to see at a specific distance. Specially designed charts other than the standard Snellen projected chart may be used.

Near Visual Acuities: Because most activities for which visually impaired patients require assistance revolve around near work, it is incumbent upon you to measure near acuity. This information will not only help the low vision therapist determine an appropriately sized target to work it, but also will help the eye care specialist to evaluate the consistency between distance and near acuity measurement.

Amber Grid Testing: It tests the central 10 degrees of vision. It can also help to determine whether the person is experiencing distortion or has (multiple) area of Scotoma.

Color Vision Testing: Several tests are available for assessing color vision. (matching or identifying yarn as in the Holmgren test). The results of this test can be held to identify the onset of a pathology, monitor a pathology, or alert the CLVT (Low Vision Therapist) to color deficits that might impact a therapeutic regimen for the patient. In addition, knowing the patient's color vision status can be important in educational, vocational, social planning or training.

Visual/Mobility Field Testing: While the patient is sitting in the chair, both monocular and binocular **confrontation fields** would be performed at 1 meter. **Perimetry Field Testing** will help evaluate the depth and breadth of an individual's peripheral vision. The visual field loss can be either absolute or relative.

Contrast Function Sensitivity Testing (CSF): It is a method of assessing the qualitative aspects of visual functioning. Two clients with the same Snellen acuity can function differently. This difference can usually be predicted with contrast sensitivity testing. It determines the client's inability to distinguish borders of a gray car against a foggy background or coffee in a dark cup.

Binocular Testing: For binocular vision to occur, the information arriving from each eye must be identical, with approximately equal vision in both eyes. To satisfy these requirements, the two eyes must be aligned so that they always point at the same object and the visual acuity, optics, or refractive errors of the two eyes must be approximately equal. This explains why, most visually impaired patients are monocular. So, this test will assess ocular alignment to determine the possibility for developing or maintaining binocular vision. A cover test and a Hirschbert test will show motor alignment. Worth Four Dot Testing will show gross fusion.

Refraction: This test will help to determine if the client has a refractive error that needs to be corrected as well as the exact lens prescription that is appropriate.

Keratometry: Will help determine the curvature of the cornea

Eye Health Evaluation: This evaluation will include but not limited to the following tests: observation of the external structures of the eye and adnexa, intraocular pressure (IOP)

measurement (tonometry) evaluation of the anterior structures of the eye, evaluation of the internal structure of the eye through a dilated pupil (unless contraindication). The purpose of this test is to determine the underlying basis for the visual acuity, contrast sensitivity and/or visual field loss. The clinician uses an ophthalmoscope to view the retina and other structures of the eye.

Magnification/Optical devices: Determining the magnification necessary for the patient to see desired materials will be important specifically in the beginning of a vision rehabilitation program. It refers to the process of enlarging the image on the retina. Magnification of an object will be accomplished by using four different methods: relative size magnification, relative distance magnification, angular magnification or electronic magnification. We will know how much magnification is needed based on the best-corrected acuities, the fields and the tasks to be address. Here, we will be able to demonstrate to the patient how the calculated magnification can be provided as a microscopy, telemicroscope, a magnifier, (stand and handheld) a projection magnifier (CCTV) or other non-optical aids and telescopes.

Other activities performed during the low vision exam: Optical devices evaluation for distance, intermediate and near vision tasks, final dispensing of devices and establishment of a follow up plan and schedule. Brightness Acuity Test (the Mentor BAT Brightness Acuity Tester can be used to subjectively determine the effect of a glare source).

What is the goal of the low exam?
The goal of the exam is to determine which devices and/or services will improve the client's use of residual vision for activities in everyday life. In other word, the goals of the low vision examination are to improve the patient's use of residual vision and to help the patient to cope better with the demands of ordinary life and, hence be independent. The low vision examination has evolved from a series of independent procedures into a structured evaluation. Each part of the sequential examination provides the clues that will help in determination of the low vision device and provide insight into success or lack of success with the low vision aid.

How is the power of a distance telescope determined?
The basic purpose of telescopic devices is to enable an individual to bring information at a distance into closer view so that objects appear larger. The Galilean telescope is often the devise selected by low vision specialists for individuals with low vision. The telescope is made of two lenses: the objective lens and the ocular lens. So, the power at which a telescope is operating is a function of the focal length of the telescope's main (objective) lens (or primary mirror) and the focal length of the eyepiece employed. The focal length of the objective lens is the distance between the lens and the point at which it brings light rays to a focus; the focal length of each eyepiece (which typically ranges from 4mm to about 40 mm) is printed on the upper surface of the eyepiece. **To calculate the power, we can just divide the focal length of the eyepiece into the focal length of the objective lens.** For example, if the Meade DS.2070AT telescope has an objective lens focal length of 700 mm; when this telescope is used with a 25 mm eyepiece, a power of 700/25 = 28 power (written as 28X) results. http://www.synapticsystems.com/sky/scopes/telbasic.html

Please note: the power of a lens is measured in diopters (D). To calculate the power of a distance of a lens in diopters (given optical infinity or light rays coming in parallel from greater than 20 feet), divide the focal distance of the lens in centimeters into 100.

D = <u>100 centimeters (40 inches)</u>

Focal distance (FD) of lens (in centimeters)

Or, the focal distance will be: 100 centimeters (40 inches)/D.

How is a magnifier (power) determined?
Magnification is the process of increasing the size of an image over a larger portion of the retina. The strength of the lenses, expressed in diopters, directly relates to the amount of magnification power an optical device has. A magnifier (power) is determined by the dividing the diopters of the lens by 4:

X magnification = D/4

Please note: the magnification power of an optical vision device is written in "X" notation, which indicates how many times the lens magnifies an image. For example: 2X, 4X, 8X.

What makes low vision exam successful for the client?

A low vision examination, often the first step in vision rehabilitation, is designed to accurately measure how one's vision works in the real world - how it functions in day-to-day living. It's not only about how well the client can see an eye chart, but also how well he/she can see faces, street signs, newspaper print, stove dials and all the other visual clues that guide you through the day. The low vision exam helps the client to use his/her functional vision more effectively. It will help determine whether special low vision optical devices, better lighting, large print reading materials or other types of training such as vision rehabilitation services, can help the individual with visual impairment to use his/her functional vision more effectively.

Another important aspect of the low vision examination is that it gives the vision professional team the information needed in order to help the client adapt emotionally to their vision loss. For example, optimal refractive correction can make a big difference in the final corrected visual acuity and visual functioning. This becomes even more important when it comes time to prescribing optical devices. Very often, we encounter patients who appear to be visually impaired or legally blind, but a **thorough refraction** indicates that the patient simply requires an updated eyeglass prescription to regain normal vision. This explains why many eye care specialists including me think that the refraction is the most important part of the low vision exam.

Low vision exam is about rehabilitation, finding new ways to accomplish the tasks of daily life- whether it's writing a grocery list, watching grandchildren play soccer or reading a menu in a restaurant.

Basic Eye Exam Components (Adults and Children):
The component of an eye exam can resume as follow:
Patient history: As in other medical specialty, an accurate history often provides a differential diagnosis upon which to base the physical examination. So, a patient history will help to determine any signs and symptoms the patient is experiencing, when they began, the presence of any general health problems, past health, allergies or medication taken, family health and eye history and occupational or environmental conditions that maybe affecting vision. For an exam, it will usually begin with the chief complaints which is characterized according to the date of onset, frequency, intermittency and duration. The location, severity and the circumstances surround onset are important as well as any associated symptoms.

Basic ophthalmologic examination or preliminary examination: This will inform on numerous variations and abnormality that occur around the eye and the eyelid. It includes **vision assessment, Visual Acuity and optical defect, measurement of glasses, accommodation, convergence, color visions, depth perception, external examinations, examinations of the ocular muscles, installation of eye drops and ointment, ophthalmoscopy, tonometry and visual field**. For example, when performing the vision assessment, the visual acuity (VA) will help evaluate how clearly each eye is seeing at distance and at near (with and without glasses). With the external examination, we will be able to evaluate the external health of the eye to determine if there any obvious abnormally related to the extra-ocular muscles, lids, cornea, pupils, conjunctiva and iris. Just a penlight will be enough to perform this exam. We will also examine the internal eye health see the lens and fundus of the eye. This would help us eliminate any possibility of the disease (like diabetic retinopathy, and, glaucoma) that may cause a vision loss. Before the refractive status of a patient is evaluated, it will be vital to know the previous prescription. This can be done with a lens meter. Using a handheld retinoscope and a lens bar, we will be able to determine any possibility of refractive errors and measurement of amplitude of accommodation. With the use of a tonometry, we will be able to check the intra-ocular pressure (IOP) of the patient...etc. With a keratometry, we will measure the curvature of the cornea, which will help determine the proper fit for contact lens. And finally, the Tests for color blindness and Depth perception will be considered. At the completion of the examination, the eye care specialist will assess and evaluate the results of the testing to determine a diagnosis and develop a treatment plan.

Based on the age of the infant, the conduct or component of **a pediatric exam** will differ. Usually the test used to evaluate child's vision (newborn to 3 years and up) are adapted for different ages and stages of development. At an early age of child development, the eye specialist needs to know how to look at responses from subjects based on age, attention span ability to point and ability to provide verbal answer. For non-verbal young children, it would be best to use the teller acuity systems (also called preferential looking testing) to determine resolution acuity at near and at intermediate distance. As I was watching the pediatric eye exam, it was great to see the different strategies used by the eye care doctor to keep the young boy engaged and motivated throughout the process. As he was more than 3 years of age and he showed adequate receptive and expressive language skills to cooperate with some of the traditional eye and vision exam. However, from time to time, the examiner needs to make modification because a child can vary significantly from expected age norms. In this way, **appropriate test procedures are often used based on child's development age and specific ability.** For example, the Lea near symbol test cannot be performed until the child reached 3-5 year of age. In the same way, the color vision testing is not effective until the child reaching the age of 3 and older.

In comparison to the traditional adult eye exam, age-appropriate examination and management strategy should be used for infant. Major modifications include relying more on objective examination procedures and performing test considerably more rapidly than with older children.

Interpreting an Eye Report
A few limitations of the eye report:
*   Information contained in the report may not be completely accurate with regard to how the individual is currently functioning or what may be expected in the future. The clinical information contained in eye report are obtained in a controlled environment with also controlled lighting along with standardized size of target. For example, the clinical visual acuity measurements do give us an approximation of the detail of the image seen at a set distance, with a set contrast and lighting, but do not give us the ability to translate this information into functional vision performance.
*   Limited testing or inadequate testing equipment. Often eye reports for younger children or individuals with multiple disabilities only mention fixation patterns such as central, steady and maintained, but offer no visual acuities. Or the report may state that the individual was difficult to test. In these cases, accurate visual acuity information will be important when determining the needs of these patients.

Content of a typical eye report:
A typical eye report includes**:**
*   Patient profile and history (which include general information, chief complaint, past health, medications and allergies, history of present illness and family history**).**
*   Visual Acuities at Near and at Distance
*   Refraction – Accommodation – Telescopic Refraction and Binocularity
*   Keratometry
*   Eye Health Examination (Lids, Conjunctiva, Cornea, Anterior Chamber, Iris and Lens)
*   Preliminary Test of Visual functions and eye health including color vision, depth perception, peripheral vision and response of the pupils to light.
*   Instillation of eye drops and ointment
*   Tonometry (I.O.P)- Ophthalmoscopy (direct and indirect)
*   Visual Fields (central and periphery)
*   Finding – Diagnosis. -RX

Define Visual Acuity. Why is the VA so important?
The visual acuity (VA) is a measure of how well an individual can see or the sharpness and clarity of an individual's vision. In other words, the VA is a measure of the smallest high-contrast detail that one can resolve. It is measured with letters or words. Usually the eye care specialist

asks the patient to read different size of letters on a chart while standing 20 feet away. The smallest letters the patient can read will be recorded as his/her acuity. The most common chart used is the Snellen Acuity Charts. It can be tested at near or at distance. The VA provides the eye care specialist with the baseline information from which the course of a pathology may be monitored. It is essential for calculating a patient's magnification needs. Inaccurate information can result in incorrect selection of optical devices for evaluation and often prolongs the duration of low vision evaluation. The determination of the VA level provides the patient with an appreciation for residual vision. In real life, its measurement helps establish eligibility for services, benefits and even driving privileges for some clients.

Description of contrast peripheral and central field testing:
A visual field test is a method of measuring an individual's entire scope of vision, that is their central and peripheral (side) vision. Visual field testing maps the visual fields of each eye individually. Usually the visual field tests are useful for detection of central or peripheral diseases affecting the visual pathways within the brain.

Clinical visual fields chart the extent of field using various testing measures including Confrontation Fields, Amsler Grid, Tangent Screen, and manual and automated perimetry techniques. Each is used for specific purposes and each yield different areas and types of visual field information.

Confrontation field testing involves the slow movement of fingers or objects from the periphery as a rough test to detect delays or gaps in response. It also requires the person to be looking straight ahead as the lights or other targets (e.g., finger puppets) are presented from various field areas. Confrontation fields provide a quick, informal check, especially for restricted peripheral fields, and are helpful for obtaining results from those who have difficulty with or are unable to respond to more formal measures.

The Amsler Grid is a chart consisting of a series of grid lines. It measures the central 10-degree field and charts the macular area responsible for detail vision.

The Tangent Screen is a black screen (e.g., black felt material) with 6 ever-widening concentric circles (outlined in white), each representing 5 degrees of central visual field. It's also tests central visual fields up to 25-30 degrees.

The Perimetry testing involve both manual and automated forms. Manual methods, not often seen today, use an arc shaped machine, where the person being tested places his or her chin in a chin rest and fixates straight ahead at the center point of the arc which rotates around a central axis. The examiner rotates the arc to cover all areas of the visual field. The Automated perimetry procedures involve the use of automated, computerized testing procedures which contribute to the reliability and validity of their results testing. The perimetry provides a more complete map of the entire visual field. Because automated perimetry techniques allow for the control of variables which impact on the extent and quality of visual field, they provide a more realistic measurement of a person's field of view.

Here are two examples: one that shows a central field loss and the other one a peripheral field loss.
- Individuals with difficulty to fixate and to see straight ahead, but where the ability to see sideways still exists. People with central field loss will belong to this group.
- Individuals with difficulties in seeing sideway but with some ability to see straight ahead. People with peripheral field loss fall under this group.

After reading the eye report, what types of questions/issues should low vision professionals raise to properly guide a thorough FVA (Functional Vision Assessment)?

Despites advancements in the accuracy and sensitivity of common visual acuity measurement in an eye report, conversion of acuity numbers into functional information, and understanding what the individual with low vision or visually impaired sees in everyday settings continue to remain an elusive task. Visual functions documented in the report, (such as visual acuity or visual field) are often measured quantitatively, have precise categories and evaluate a single variable at a time. Tests of visual functions are usually performed in a static environment with controlled lighting, standardized size targets, and high contrast targets. By contrast, functional vision assessment in an eye report should describe how the individual functions and should also involve measure of the individual's visual skills and abilities as applied to performance of usual tasks of daily life, such as reading. Very often, functional vision is described qualitatively. It should be measured binocularly to replicate the individual's visual performance in the real world and examines supra-threshold performance so that the individual's comfort level for an activity could be identified. An evaluation of functional vision should be affected by multiple variable at one time. Functional vision evaluation is usually performed in dynamic environments. **In this way, the information contained in a medical eye report could raise many questions about the accuracy of how the individual is currently functioning.** For example, in some cases, parents of a children with visual impairment may be told their children are blind, or will become blind, without being giving additional explanation about the effects of the child's conditions on visual functioning or its likely progression.

Chapter 7:
Special Considerations-Questions/Answers
1. Ergonomic Positions and Visual Performance
2. Prism and Functional Visual Assessment
3. Low Vision and Adaptive Diabetes Self-management
4. Developing Effective Communication Skills to Stay Connected with Friends and Relatives
5. A Visually Impaired Client in A Shopping Center
6. The AZOOR (Acute Zonal Occult Outer Retinopathy)

1. **Ergonomic positions and Visual Performance**

Comfortable working posture (ergonomic positions) is an important factor that can influence the visual performance of our clients. To quote Chris Newton from the Eastern Blin Rehab Center (EBRC), CT, VA:" *Anytime a client is in an unstable position, he/she may feel insecure and will be unable to concentrate on the task. The priority should always be postural security"*. Although it can be very challenging for someone with visual impairments or with other physical disabilities to hold his/her body upright and demonstrate effective visual response, he/she will do it with good practice. During my internship at the EBRC, I had one-hour session training with a Veteran concentrated on ergonomic position in the beginning of a Video Magnifier (CCTV) training. During the reading training with recommended near lenses, I realized that he should be free of any physical stress of maintaining his balance to sustain visual attention.

Please see below a few tips developed by Yates (1989) to help clients diagnosed with multiple disabilities:
- Client should be positioned in a way that does not reinforce an abnormal muscle pattern
- Client should have support where it is necessary, but not at the expense of voluntary freedom of movement
- Client should be visually symmetrical and should not be leaning off-center.... etc.

All the above explain why Vision Rehab Specialists often recommend reading stand or lap desk to their clients.

2. **Prism and Functional Visual Assessment**

Generally, the prism causes a displacement of an object in the patient's blind area to an area on the retina where there is useful vision. In other word, the prism is placed on the area of the yet that is non-seeing and therefore does not cause an additional blind spot or dual image.

Among the different type of prism, the Fresnel prism is the most commonly used for field enhancement. The Fresnel Prism is a 1.mm plastic (poly vinyl chloride) material that can initially be placed on the outer edge of both spectacle lenses (base out) so the individual can make small eye movements into the prism to check for objects in the peripheral (65 to 85 degrees). This eliminates the need for inefficient net movements to accomplish the same task. The person becomes more aware of objects in the peripheral once he/she learns to scan systematically into the prism (Randall Jose, Understand Low Vision, page 367).

Journal article search – What does the literature say?

As Fresnel Prism were evaluated, prescribed and reported in the literature, it became evident that not all peripheral defects responded equally. According to Brilliant R., the successful cases were with those patients having a hemianopic field loss and the most success was with bitemporal hemianopic field loss. In these cases, prisms placed base out at the temporal aspect of the carrier lenses were well received. It has become apparent that not all peripheral field defects are sensitive to the same methods of field enhancement. For example, patient with gradual field loss may learn to be more efficient with their scanning ability and therefore have less need for prisms or mirrors.

The Pros and Cons of using prism for VFE, and how they play a role in VFE assessment:

Therapeutic prisms, based on the principle of Fresnel, when compared with conventional prisms, have been shown to be superior cosmetically and more adaptable therapeutically because of the reduced weight and thickness. Functionally, however, the Press On membrane prism shows deficiencies which limit its usefulness in the higher powers required for prismotherapy. For this group of patients, a "perfected wafer" like the hard prism of the Fresnel prism trial set, would be acceptable prisms for therapeutic use.

The advantage of the Fresnel prism is that it is inexpensive lighter (minimal weight) and can be easily changed as the person's ability to scan improves (It has a wide range of available power from 0.5 prism diopters to 30 prism diopters).

However, the Fresnel prisms have some disadvantages
- They can cause blurry vision when the person views through it
- They can cause a decrease in contrast sensitivity at all spatial frequencies and especially at the high spatial frequencies.
- The prisms will discolor overtime and may lose the surface tensions over a period and fall off.
- They demonstrate greater distortion and chromatic aberrations than an equal-powered ground-in prism.

Although the ophthalmic sector prisms are more expensive, but it provides better clarity, durability and peripheral vision performance than the plastic prism. The ophthalmic sector prisms give the person a clear image when viewing through it, but it cannot be modified. Experience shows that the blurred image or slight haziness from the Fresnel system and the cost of the ophthalmic system are the most often report reasons for people not proceeding with the treatment option. So, the Fresnel prism are not recommended for the high functioning hemianopsia patients especially if driving is a consideration owing to the need for higher contrast.

The observation of all the above factors led to the development of new clinical protocol knowing as peripheral field awareness system than as a field – enhancement system as would be the case with reverse telescope. The protocol combined the advantages of both types of prism to better assist patients. The new protocol would help fit the person initially with the Fresnel prism, with the intent of moving to ophthalmic prism as the final prescription. So, it is important to explain that blurring is a characteristic of Fresnel prism but that it can be eliminated with a more expensive ophthalmic prism, after it has been determined that the prism system will benefit the person's ability to travel independently.

3. **Low vision and adaptive diabetes Self-management**

According to researchers at the Center for Disease Control and Prevention and the U.S. Census Bureau, the prevalence of diabetes and vision loss have been increased in the past years as the result of the aging population and the rising incidence of obesity along with stress related issues. As of 2010, statistic reports from the American Diabetes Association (ADA) revealed that 20.8 million people in the United States or 7 % of the population are affected by either Type I (Insulin-dependent) or Type II (non-insulin dependent) diabetes.

Generally, control of diabetes involves maintaining near normal blood glucose levels through diet; exercise; and for many, medication including insulin. Nearly 86% of those who have had diabetes for more than 15 years will experience some form of vision loss and many will become severely visually impaired (ADA, 2010). Because the prevalence of diabetes cases related to vision loss is increasing, Vision Rehabilitation Professionals will be more frequently called to assist such individuals with the tasks involved in managing their condition. As a Vision Rehabilitation Professional, we must be familiar with diabetes and its management. It is the role of the Physician, Nurse or Diabetes Educator to provide treatment and instruction about the controlling diabetes. Vision Rehabilitation Professionals are often the source of information and provide instruction regarding techniques and adaptive devices for measuring insulin and blood glucose levels (*Ponchillia, 1996*) for clients with diabetes and visual impairments.

This week, July 29th – 30th, I had the opportunity to attend a "Low vision and adaptive diabetes self-management course at the Salus University by the Diabetes Educator Debra Sokol-Mckay. Unfortunately, I did not obtain any essential information that could help me better understand diabetes or any new adaptive skills that I could use to assist my future clients. There are so many devices out there that are available for clients and the focus of the class was only on the device "*Prodigy*". During the two days of classes, I had to reflect on my own knowledge and experience to be able to assist others.

So, based on the outline of the class, I had to develop my own knowledge such as:

A. **Environmental modifications**: This involves good lighting, organization skills, contrast sensitivity and magnification.

The amount of light reflected from the surface of the viewed blood glucose device into the client's eye will be critical for visibility. Generally, as the degree of illumination is increased so is visibility- at least, up to a point. Therefore, one of the first assessments a Vision Rehabilitation professional will make in a client's home is the adequacy of the lighting. Very often, for low vision clients, a simple addition of lights along with increase contrast between the adaptive insulin device (Count – a-dose or syringe support) and the background of the tray with the required materials can improve their visibility. After the first day of the class, I had the opportunity to teach my nephew some of the basic adaptive tasks that will help him monitor his blood glucose.

My nephew is 28 years old and has been diagnosed with diabetes Type I since he was 10 years old. Recently his vision started deteriorated and is unable to monitor his blood sugar the way he used to do. His last eye exam revealed a VA 20/600 OD, 20/400 OS and 5-degree field of view. He wanted to monitor the level of his blood glucose safely and independently. In order to assist him, I required the following materials:

- Blue tray (Available at Amazon. Item# 40098. Price: $15.18)
- Blood glucose monitor with speech output. (Available at Save Rite Medical. Item# 56-7151. Price: $43.20. His health insurance pays for it)
- Gauze, alcohol swab, and glove. (Available at his house)
- Logbook (or Standard Pilot Logbooks. Available at Amazon.com. Item # ASA-SP-57. Price: $11.95.
- Syringe, reagent strip, spring-loaded lancet device, and sharp container. Source: CVS and paid by his health insurance.
- Hand sanitizer. (Available at Market Lab. Item # #ML1258. Price: $ 36:00

In a large open space (900 sq. ft.) with bright fluorescent lights and floor carpeted in brown, my nephew learned to do the following tasks:

- Assemble the desirable equipment and supplies (reagent strips, loaded lancet syringe and syringe support, blood glucose monitor with speech output, alcohol pad and hand sanitizer) required for the test and place them in memorable positions on the blue tray while using the clock face as guide direction.
- Practice in locating and identifying each one of the materials on the tray without any accidents occurring.
- Locate the hand sanitizer in your tray and clean your hands prior to performing the test
- Keep your hands below the heart to increase the blood flow
- Use your dominant hand to locate ¼ part of the distal (outward) side of the finger for lancing
- Milk the finger down its length toward the tip to format enough blood droplet. Count the number of times the finger is milked to produce a hanging drip
- Lance the finger near the monitor so the blood sample is not likely jolted off while moving the finger toward the targeted area.

- Lance the finger on the outside and touching only the drop of blood to the trip
- Angle the machine so that the hand can reach out at is natural angle to deposit the blood on the strip placed in the machine.
- Used landmark on the machine such as straight or curved parts locate the target area
- Listen attentively to obtain the result of the blood glucose level.
- Record the test score in his booklet

My nephew will continue to perform the tasks until he has mastered the above skills. In addition, as a Vision Rehabilitation Professional, we must know that managing diabetes involves a balance of diet, exercise and medicine (insulin or oral agents) as well as daily blood glucose (sugar) monitoring to better assist our clients. If this balance is kept, it can avoid long-term problems caused by diabetes.

Personal Observation –
After the above session training, I realized the vision rehabilitation professionals must be well prepared and ready to help the physicians, nurses and diabetes educators to control any variable that may interfere with success. We must be prepared to teach some adaptive techniques to better assist our clients. For example, using a small plastic pipette to gather blood and disperse it on the targeted area may assist clients who have difficulty getting the blood on the strip.

In addition, some glucose monitors are very often fitted with attachments to help aim the blood onto the strip.
   A. **Adaptation for**: Proper strip orientation, test strip insertion, location of blood sample on finger and apply blood to test site. Here again, vision rehabilitation can educate clients on some adaptive techniques to locate and perform the diabetes tasks. They can teach them landmark on the device, such as **raised dots or other tactile or contrasting markings.**
   B. **Insulin Pumps:** There are different kinds of insulin pumps in the market. We must know the basic information about how to make them better serve our clients. Vision rehabilitation professional must understand that the insulin pumps do not check blood glucose. It's another way our clients get steady flow of insulin.

4. **"Developing effective communication skills to stay connected with friends and relatives".**
A practicing Vision Rehabilitation Therapist likely uses just about every medium to communicate with his/her clients. We talk on the phone, send email messages, converse one on one, participate in meetings and verbal/written recommendations. Although *"active listening"* is the starting place for effective communication, helping clients with visual impairment to maintain their address books or list of telephone numbers up to date and legible is important to enable them to stay in communication with their loved ones.

My mother is 74 years old and lives by herself in her own apartment in Brooklyn, New York. In the past few weeks, she has experienced a decrease of her vision and photophobia during her daily living activities. Recently, she has been diagnosed with severe glaucoma in both eyes. She has difficulty to do the following tasks at near distance:

- Reading phone numbers from her address book
- Writing checks to pay her bills

In addition to the above concerns, she wants to be able to maintain a list of telephone numbers to stay in communication with friends and relatives.

To help her out, I decided to teach her writing techniques along with other alternative techniques for keeping her telephone list.

1. **Materials or adapted writing tools used**:
   - Bold lined paper or paper with extra bold lines
   - Dark felt tip pens, markers, the Sanford 20/20 Easy-to-Read Pen
   - Writing guides (Signature, envelop and check writing guides in addition to handwriting grids)
   - Task lighting (gooseneck lamp which shines directly on the writing area
   - Dark colored clipboard

Since she has lost her vision, no simulator- glasses were used for learning activities. The above well-contrasted materials prevent glare and allowed her to see lined paper and read bold numbers using the felt-tip pen. With practices, she will be able to independently sign her name, address an envelope, and write a check for her electricity bill. Experiences shows that the "older people may manage to write, take notes and write down telephone numbers but cannot read back what he/she has written" (*Orr, A., 2003*). This situation was different for my mother case. Writing with the dark felt tip pens along with the extra bold lines made it easier for her to read back what she had written.

Before the end of the training, she was evaluated on the following skills:
- Finding the line which to sign or writing (5)
- Knowing the proper amount of space to sign or write in (5)
- Keeping the bases of the letters on the bases
- Maintaining proper letter spacing (5)
- Highlight all her friends and relatives phone numbers from her address book (5)
- Find her close friends phone number from her address book to call (5)
- Add and remove phone numbers from her address book (5)

Her final score: 30/30 (5+5+5+5+5+5)
Although, she was happy for being able to achieve her goals, I did verbally educate her on some alternative technique for keeping her telephone list such as cassette recoding of the telephone list, including important names and numbers. CCTV was also recommended.

5. **A Visually Impaired Client in a Shopping Center**

Generally, when buying some things at a shopping center or restaurant or even paying for a movie ticket or for a new pair of shoes, we always make sure that we are handing the seller the right amount. This is simple, we just have to give a quick look at our money, take out the right amount, and that's it. However, for someone who is blind or visually impaired, distinguishing among bills of different denominations and determining the authenticity of the bill can be difficult or impossible. The vision rehabilitation professional should be aware of the right techniques in order to help clients satisfy their needs.

Early this morning (7-12-2015: 2:45 PM), I simulated the vision of my 35-year-old female medical examiner to a total loss with a blindfold. The simulation was performed in the waiting area of Express Health Services (Valley Stream, NY) with bright large fluorescent lighting.

As goal, she wanted to be able to provide the correct amount of money when making a purchase.

Objective: At the end of the training, when making a purchase, she will be familiar with a system for identifying bills and differentiating among coins tactilely.

Materials needed for the training:
- Different types of coins, dime, quarter, penny, nickel and dollars bills ($5, $10 and $20)
- Blindfold
- Table, adjustable chairs.
- Lighting

Before beginning the training, I handed her different coins and bills for exploration and familiarization. It was important that she demonstrated the ability to identify her money by:
- Consistently identifying each coin correctly
- Differentiating bills using a consistent effective method

Because she was blindfolded, she was unable to see the difference in color between the copper penny and the other silver coins. So, I had her develop specific cues for differentiating coins:
- Size - The dime is the smallest
- Thickness - The nickel is the thickest
- Edges – the penny and nickel have smooth edges and the dime, and the quarter have grooved edges

The following **steps** for training where performed:
1. Layout coins. Place the penny, nickel, dime and quarter in her hand one at a time. We did not practice with a dollar coin however; she will practice when that coin is available.
2. Feel the coins. Finger the coins and observe the size edges and thickness of them.
3. Try to identify coins that you are to distinguish
4. Practice. At this step in the training, I worked with her to identify the coins that she was unable to identify by using the size, edges and thickness cue.

When it comes to bills, the task was easier. She knew about the folding technique when she was in Nursing School. After observing her methods, I advised her to continue using it. To refresh her knowledge, I had her performed the following:
- Leave the $1-dollar bills unfolded or flat in her purse
- Fold the $5-dollar bills end to end (square shaped)
- Fold the $10-dollar bills in half lengthwise (long narrow rectangle shaped)
- Fold the $20-dollar bill in quarter sections. Similar to the $5-fold but fold it again

Adaptations:
Before the end of training, I advised her to purchase a wallet or billfold with several different slots or pockets for sorting coins and bills. When purchasing, try to use bills and coins that are as close to the purchase price as possible. This might avoid her to sort and identify her change when returning home.

She was also advised on the following (as needed):
- Use the assistance of trusted sighted individuals
- Use of affordable electronic talking identifier money device
- Always count bills at the crease, note where both edges of the bills come together
- Refer her to an elementary math curriculum for skills in calculating change or the use of a talking calculator.

Personal Observation:
During the training lesson, it's amazing to see how important it might be for a client to be able to handle his/her money and make purchases independently. It can be difficult for a client with visual impairment to tell different denominations of money apart, especially bills, but there are systems available to make this much easier. When shopping, it might be helpful that clients give no larger combination of bills and coins than necessary in order to avoid receiving a large amount of change. This habit will reduce the chances of receiving incorrect change and mixing up one's remaining money.

6. **The AZOOR (Acute Zonal Ocult Outer Retinopathy). – Questions/Answers**

Understanding the AZOOR Disease

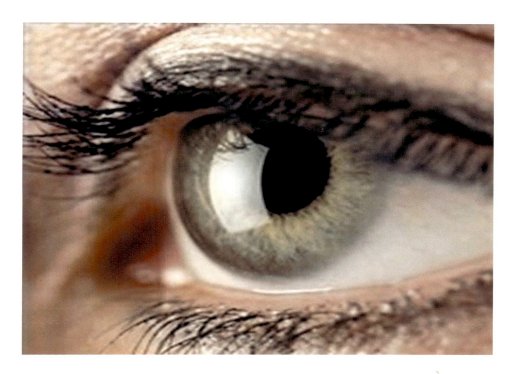

Azoor eye disease also known as *"acute zonal occult retinopathy"*, a rare eye disease which is characterized by sudden onset of retina inflammation and could lead to blindness. As named, AZOOR is a unique disease characterized by zonal patches of inflammation within the outer retina associated with minimal changes on fundus examination (Gass, 1992). The AZOOR affects mainly young women and often characterized by white/gray dots at the level of the retinal pigment epithelium, vitreous cells and transient electoretinographics abnormalities. To understand the AZOOR disease it is important to master the major parts of the eye (specifically the retina), where the visual information is collected and transmitted. A thorough foundation on the anatomy-physiology of the retina will enable us to better understand the functional and educational implications by this disease.

The Retina and Optic Nerve Head

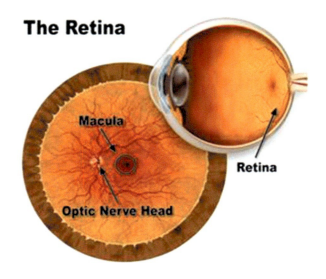

The Retina is the most internal coat of the eye. It is a thin delicate membrane with ten distinct layers of cells. It contains the sensory receptors for the transmissions of light. The retinal receptors are divided in two main populations: **rods** (function best in dim light) and **cones** (functions well under daylight conditions, color vision). The cones form a concentrated area in the retina known as the Fovea, which lies in the center of the macula. Whenever we look at an object, we must aim the eye so that the image of the object is focused on the Fovea. Smooth eye movement called pursuits and jump eye movements, called saccades are both designed to allow people to use the Fovea. So, the Retina serves to receive visual images and transmit information to the optical pathways of the brain through the optic nerve. In this way, light may pass through all layers of the retina to reach the photoreceptors where the visual process begins. Diseases like macular degeneration, AZOOR or diabetic retinopathy that affect the clarity of retina, or swelling that affects the shape of the retina, will have a profound effect on vision.

The Macula
- Is the thinnest part of the retina
- The fovea, the center of the macula, provides the 20/20 acuity
- Is not fully developed until about 6 months or so after birth

Functions:
- Receives light
- Transmits light
- Converts light to visual energy

Reflection on functions of the 10 layers of the retina:
The retina is a specialized neural tissue that lines the back of the eye. This tissue is responsible for capturing light and converting it to a chemical signal. There are ten layers of the retina and each serves a specific purpose in order to enable a person to see colors.

Retinal Pigmented Epithelium (RPE): is the last layer of the retina. It's a highly pigmented layer that absorbs excess light. The RPE serves as a nourishing and garbage –collecting layer for the photoreceptors. Its cells have very tight junctions between themselves, which prevent diffusion of substances between the choroidal circulation and the retina. This is the last layer of the retina and is attached to the structures behind the retina.

Photoreceptor: these are the rods and cones that receive light and undergo a chemical configuration change to detect light.

External Limiting Membrane: represents where the inner segments of the rods and cones are located. It's formed from adherens junctions between Muller cells and photoreceptor cell inner segments. It also forms a barrier between the sub retinal space, into which the inner and outer segments of the photoreceptors project to be in close association with the pigment epithelial layer behind the retina, and the neural retinal proper.

Outer Nuclear layer (ONL): these are the actual cell bodies of the rods and cones. It's about the same thickness in central peripheral retina. However, in peripheral rod, cell bodies outnumber the cone cell bodies which the reverse is true for central retina.

Outer Synaptic Layer or Outer Plexiform Layer (OPL): These are where the projections from the rods and cones synapse with the bipolar cells.

Inner Nuclear Layer (INL): contains the nuclei of the bipolar cells, horizontal and amacrine cells. The bipolar cells are responsible for relaying information from the photoreceptors to the ganglions.

Inner Synaptic Layer or Inner Plexiform Layer (IPL): is the area where the bipolar cells axons and the dendrites of the ganglion cells synapse. This area is where the two cells communicate. This is the area where the message concerning the visual image is transmitted to the brain along with the optic nerve.

Ganglion Cell Layer: contains nuclei of ganglion cells, the axons of which become the optic nerve fibers for messages and some amacrine cells. These ganglion cells are vital for transmitting the information from the photoreceptors to the brain. Damage to these cells will cause loss of vision.

Nerve Fiber Layer: is comprised of the axons of the ganglion's cells. Loss of nerve fibers can cause loss of vision, generally of the peripheral visions first before the central vision.

Internal Limiting Membrane: is the first structure light hits. It is the basement membrane for a cell called the Muller cell. The Muller cells serve as supporting structures for retinal ganglion cell complex. It is the inner surface of the retina forming a diffusion barrier between neural retina and vitreous humor.

Central and peripheral retina compared.
Central retina close to the fovea is considerably thicker than peripheral retina. This is due to the increased packing density of photoreceptors, particularly the cones, and their associated bipolar and ganglion cells in central retina compared with peripheral retina. **The Central retina is cone-dominated retina whereas peripheral retina is rod-dominated**.

Rods and Cones

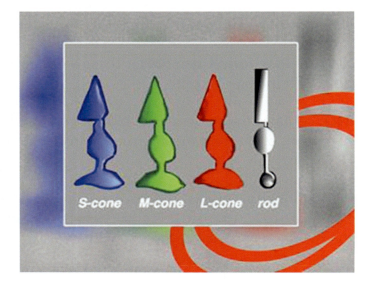

Rods and cones are specialized nerve cells. They contain an outer segment, which is sensitive to light, and an inner segment, which is similar to a typical axon or inner portion of a nerve cell.

Rods

The rods allow us to see at night and to perceive motion. The visual discrimination is of rods is not very high. They function in scotopic conditions (low illumination). There are no rods in the macular area. Hundreds of rods connect (converge) through the bipolar and the other middle cells before connecting to a few ganglions. This allows our side vision to act as the travel vision. The rods function in scotopic conditions and provide vision in shades of gray.

Cones

Cones provide our detailed, color and phototropic (bright light) vision. There are approximately 6 to 8 million cones in the retina. Cones are the only photoreceptors in the foveola. There is a one-to-one connection of cones to ganglion cells in the retina. This is why the macular has such accurate and detailed vision. The cones are tightly packed together in the macular area. Cones are less light sensitive, requiring more light to be stimulated.

Cones also consist of an outer segment, nucleus and inner segment. The visual pigment of the cones is contained in discs in the outer segment of the cones. Cones have three visual pigments:
   • Erythrolabe: Red catching
   • Chlorolabe: Green catching
   • Cyanolabe: Blue catching

The combination of red, green and blue cones contributes to our perception of color.
All the above to say, based on the components of the Retina affected, the clinical presentations of the AZOOR will be different from. This also explains why the management of the disease is different from one patient to another. Although the success of all the researches performed

eye care institutes, universities and independents Eye care specialists, the etiology of AZOOR is as yet, unknown and the nature of the associations between the dysfunction and uni or multifocal inflammation have not been also identified. It is an unpredictable, often disabling disease of the retinal structure that disrupts the flow of visual information between the eye and the brain. The progress, severity and specific symptoms of AZOOR are limited in space and time. In other words, there are a variety of presenting signs and symptoms in AZOOR that involve many different areas of the retinal structure, and the inability to attribute them all to one localizing lesions is a characteristic feature of the disease.

However, many researches performed by eye care specialists postulate the following causes: infection (viral), autoimmune disease, or non-disease specific genetic background, inflammatory and some exogenous agents.

Generally, patients diagnosed with AZOOR are women who present with acute unilateral visual disturbances, often following a viral illness.

Commons signs and symptoms and mechanisms:
The symptomatology of the disease varies from patient to patient:
- Presence of blind spot spanning in peripheral area of vision and more noticeable in natural light.
- Variable color visions in a dim area
- Photophobia: car – headlights at night can be almost debilitating and when the sun shines on the snow.
- Usually the retinal lesions gradually regress with time leaving only minor retinal pigment epithelial defects.

Although the above signs and symptoms are not specific to AZOOR, their presence are due to some form of defect of the photoreceptors of the retina **(Rods and Cones)**. Remember the rods are in the peripheral retina and allow us to see at night and perceive motion. They allow our side visions to act as the travel vision. They function in scotopic conditions and provide vision in shades of gray. In the other hand, the cones are represented by the pneumonic **3C**, which stand for **Color, Contrast and Clarity**. The cones are less light sensitive and often require more light to be simulated.

There seems to be overlap between AZOOR and other eye conditions like MEWDS (Multiple Evanescent White Dot Syndrome), AMN (Acute Macular Neuro-retinopathy), Birdshot Chorio-retinopathy, Serpiginous choroidopathy, AMPPE and the entities of multifocal choroiditis (MFC), Diffuse subretinal fibrosis syndrome and punctuate inner choroidopathy (PIC), each being a different manifestation of similar Pathophysiological processes.

The diagnostic of choice is usually made by electroretinogram which will indicate the field loss due to retinal dysfunction. In AZOOR, retinal dysfunction is usually occurring without corresponding visible retinal lesions.

There is no cure for AZOOR. Most of the treatment options envisaged by eye care specialists only help to relieve symptoms of acute exacerbations and prevent relapses. Based on the conditions that lead to AZOOR, Eye care specialists consider the following treatments:

- Immunosuppressant
- Steroid
- PDT or anti-VEGF Therapy if there is a choroidal neovascularized
- Antivirals or antifungal etc.

During the last 6 months, I worked with 2 Veteran diagnosed with AZOOR. They went to all types of surgery at the Wilmer Eye Institute with no improvement. It took them over 2 years to decide to see a low vision specialist. At the VA in Connecticut, they were able to learn visual skills along with other techniques that help them use efficiently the remaining of their visions. They were able to use optical and non- optical devices recommended safety and independently for their daily living activities. To quote one of them at the end of the program: *"The bigger mistake I made in my life it listened to my wife and my retinal specialist Doctor. I should have listened to my gut and come here sooner. "*

Chapter 8:
Psych-Social Consequences of Visual Impairment

It is important to keep in mind that the loss of vision extends into several different areas and that meaning, and extent of each loss varies for each individual. We need to understand how each area has been impacted upon.

The following losses are highlighted to have us start to think about the pervasiveness of loss and change provoked by visual impairment:

1. **Loss of mobility:**
   - Change in independence
   - Loss of travel options
   - Loss of social contacts
   - Overall change in level of activity
   - Loss of feeling of security and safety

2. **Loss of activities of daily living:**
   - Loss of control over the environment
   - Fear of displacement (e.g., being forced to move in with a relative, moving to a nursing home)
   - Changes in roles and responsibilities
   - Change in self-esteem due to inability to care for oneself and one's home

3. **Loss of communication:**
Written:
   - Loss of privacy (e.g., having mail read by others, turning over personal finances to others)
   - Loss of control (e.g., having someone else pick out a greeting card)
   - Loss of access to written news, current events

Nonverbal:
   - Loss of ability to experience nonverbal communication (e.g., facial expression, body language)
   - May lead to avoidance of social situations

4. **Loss of avocation (Leisure activities)**
   - Loss of self-fulfillment: May lead to stagnation, depression and decrease in social contacts especially significant for older adults who may fill time with leisure activities

5. **Loss of career/vocational goal/opportunities**
   - Loss or change in job may lead to changes in self-esteem, feelings of productivity and self-worth
   - May also have financial ramifications and well as lead to role change within the family unit

6. **Loss of independence**
   - Ties in with all the potential losses
   - May be a struggle between the desire for independence and its freedom and the desire for dependence and its protection
   - Degree of the impact of this loss connected to personality

7. **Loss of obscurity**
   - Loss of ability to blend in, feel part of the "crowd"
   - May impact on willingness to use adaptive equipment in public (e.g., large print, low vision devices, white cane)
   - Increased feeling of vulnerability
   - Issues with having a reference group with whom to compare self

8. **Loss of sexuality**
   - May no longer feel attractive or desirable
   - Ties in with changes in self-image, self-concept
   - Feedback from others is critical
   - Partner may feel inhibited—unsure how to react or respond

9. **Loss of spontaneity**
   - Loss of freedom to come and go as one pleases
   - Increased dependency on others
   - Loss of control over planning one's time

Internal factors in the adjustment Process/Passing Behavior:
Generally, the term passing is defined as a cultural performance whereby one member of a defined social group masquerades as another in order to enjoy the privileges afforded to dominant group. In other words, passing is simply choosing not to disclose one's invisible stigma in order to appear to be part of the dominant or not stigmatized group. A person with visual impairment may choose to use this behavioral strategy to achieve a specific goal. To quote Irving Goffman "passing refers to when *the person chooses to conceal a salient aspect of who he/she is to preserve one's sense of self*".

1. **Description of a situation in which a person with visually impairment might choose to pass and discuss how internal factors affecting adjustment influence this choice:**
An 80-year-old woman with age related macular disease who refused to read any passage in the bible at church to prevent being excluded from her singing group activities. She tries to pass as a sighted individual at the church and doesn't want her peers to know about her

vision problem. So, when she is at church with her peers whose attitudes towards blindness or visually impaired are unknown, she is frequently tempted to withhold the information that she is visually impaired. When there is a church group activity, she pretends to be sighted and goes with the flow. Very often, she relinquishes her own personal attributes, aspirations, standards and values to adopt her peer's ones in order to comply with their activities. In this situation, the 80-year-old woman has not accepted her vision impairment as one of her personal characteristics along with all the others. There is a serious blow to her self-esteem and her feeling of self-worth, ability and significance. (*Coopersmith, 1967*). She creates a false identity in order to avoid revealing her stigmatized trait. In situations, internal factors affecting adjustment may influence the following:

- Her current state of physical well-being
- Her typical or patterned responses to changes, stress or crisis
- The presence or absence of other health conditions
- Religious and cultural beliefs

2. **What are the potential risks and benefits of the "passing" behavior?**

As far as potential risks, individuals who choose to use passing behavior will need to constantly aware of social cues in order to avoid accidentally disclosing information about their hidden identity, a worry that most individuals from dominant group do not share. As well documented above, individuals who use this behavior have a potential risk of losing their own personal attributes, aspirations, standards, interest and values to adopt someone else's.

As a vision rehabilitation professional, it would be important to understand that. In other words, they are at risk of losing **internal perceptions of** self. (Self-concept). They may be at risk of losing the ability to adapt to social and physical requirements of the environment (*Tuttle & Tuttle, page 57*). For example, the 80-year-old woman mays reject assistance for the following key reasons:

- Fear of admitting that she has a vision problem and that she needs assistance to read passages on her bible at church.
- Loss of self-esteem or self-confidence or feeling of uselessness and worthlessness...etc.

The **main issue t**hat can arise from passing is that the individuals feel as though they are not true to themselves, which can create an inner sense of turmoil and lead to psychological strain for the person hiding their identity. This can lead to a myriad of negative workplace consequences including job satisfaction, less organizational commitment, strained social relationship and higher turnover intentions.

As far as benefits of the passing behavior, it helps the person enjoy the privileges afforded to the dominant group.

3. **How could you as a professional working with students/clients or patients help to address the situation?**

Adjusting to vision loss is a sequential process, which follows the same pattern, or phases, as that of adjusting to any of life's many traumas or crises. Our role should be to **teach technical**

skills that could help accommodate with the vison loss and assist through the phase of adjustment. When working with client(s), it would be essential to have some level of awareness and an appreciation for the range of emotions experienced by the individual experienced the vision loss. We must share insight and offer support to them. The ability and willingness to recognize and respond to their emotional needs while working with them, might make the vision care much more effective and ultimately contribute to a higher level of their satisfaction with the vision rehabilitation services. The used of Active listening techniques might lead to a better understanding of his/her feeling. Through this process, a trusting relationship could be established, and more effective services will be able to provide.

Negativism and depression have a way of perpetuating themselves. So, we will need to work with the client who is blind or visually impaired **to redirect thought patterns onto the good and positive and redirect mental energies toward setting realistic goals, developing social contacts and other appropriate activities.**

One of the negative consequences of passing is strained social relationship with peers, coworkers and friends. Therefore, **disclosure** can have a substantial impact on well-being as a result of obtaining social support. In other words, receiving positive reactions from interaction partners through disclosure can lead to positive outcome in a daily living environment.

Chapter 9:
Living Skills Cases

Food Preparation and Daily Living skills – Lesson Plans

Today many homemakers who are visually impaired or blind can cook, sew, clean the house and raise a family with no more difficulty than a sighted person. These individuals learn appropriate safety techniques from highly experienced Vision Rehabilitation Professionals. The activities of daily living (ADL) encompass an enormous range of behaviors, from brushing one's teeth, fixing a leaky faucet, and preparing/eating a meal, etc. Learning skills in the area of food preparation can be an important piece that can reinforce skills like organization, fine motor, and follow directions. The nice thing about learning techniques like spreading, measuring, pouring and chopping is that each technique can broadens with a client's choice of meals.

1. **Background**: Early this morning (10-7-2019: 9:45 AM to 11:00 AM), I had the opportunity to instruct Mr. Richard on some adaptive kitchen skills. He is a 36-year-old Caucasian male diagnosed with glaucoma OU and diabetes retinopathy OS. His visual acuity was 10/40 OD, 10/50+ OS. His goal was to be able to appropriately use nested measuring cups and spoons when making his favor meal (**oatmeal)**.

LESSON OBJECTIVE: Adaptive kitchen skills - Measuring ingredients - When presented with nested measuring cups the client will be able to measure ingredients for a recipe without any mistakes.

Materials needed for the training: graduated measuring cups, mixing bowl, water table knife, spoon, lighting and a well-contrasted (blue) tray.

Mixing - The student will be able to mix recipe ingredients until well blended.

STEPS TAUGHT/INSTRUCTION PROVIDED: Mr. Richard was provided adaptive labeling techniques for labeling a Pyrex measuring container, measuring cups, and measuring spoons. As a CVRT (Certified Vision Rehabilitation Therapist), I provided adaptive measuring techniques for measuring dry and liquid ingredients. Adaptive mixing techniques were also discussed.

SUCCESS OF INSTRUCTION: Mr. Richard was able to use the techniques shown to successfully measure and mix the correct amounts of dry and liquid ingredients to prepare a beverage mixture of Crystal Light Iced Tea. He did have difficulty opening the plastic package of powder and had to use his teeth. In this situation, I informed him that he could have also used scissors to open the package. He was satisfied with the product. He reported that he could use the techniques shown to label measuring devices at home to make them accessible to him.

BARRIERS (IF ANY): Limited hand dexterity

CLEARANCE/SAFETY ISSUES (IF ANY): Potential safety concerns were discussed and shown using scissors for opening food packaging.

NEXT CLASS OBJECTIVE: Continue with adaptive kitchen skills; Cutting, Chopping, Slicing, Dicing, Peeling - He will be able to peel various vegetables and chop them into bite sized pieces without any complications.

2. **Background: Mr. Fritz is a** 59-year-old Spanish American male, diagnosed with Stargardt' disease OU and his blindness is due to maculopathy. He is currently having the following recommended devices: OD: -4.25 -3.50 X 010, OS: -4.25 -4.00 X 160, illuminated handheld magnifier 6.5 X / 22D PWR MAG SPT and monocular telescope PD 36, 38 OS. CCTV SRX OD: -1.75 -3.50 X 010 OS: -1.75 -4.00 X 160 5D LUXO LAMP with +10D Loupe, Floor Stand, and Casters.

His goals were to be able to prepare breakfast safely and independently when his Home Health Aid is not available.

LESSON OBJECTIVE: Meal preparation using the microwave, handling and transferring hot foods, adaptive timing, and monitoring doneness.

Materials needed: microwave machine, bread, bacon, egg, tray, plate, spoon, fork, knife, coffee mug, timer (Reizen talking timer), lighting and doneness

INSTRUCTION PROVIDED: First, I provided an orientation on the microwave and discussed appropriate cooking times for common items. Adaptive seasoning techniques were shown as well as handling hot foods, cleanup prevention, and cleanup. He was shown how to use the microwave to prepare breakfast food (egg and bacon).

SUCCESS OF INSTRUCTION: Mr. Fritz was able to successfully use the microwave to cook scrambled eggs in a coffee mug. He was also able to prepare bacon. He was able to select the appropriate cooking times for each item, and monitor doneness by using texture, sound, and smell.

BARRIERS (IF ANY): Limited hand dexterity – Mr. Fritz had difficulty handling utensils and transferring foods in and out of the microwave.

CLEARANCE/SAFETY ISSUES (IF ANY): Safety concerns include the possibility of spilling hot foods on self and dropping items.

NEXT CLASS OBJECTIVE: Adaptive stove safety techniques. He will be able to locate burners and center pan. Stovetop safety and controls will be introduced.

3. **Background**: **Mr. Fritz is a** 59-year-old Spanish American male, diagnosed with Stargardt' disease OU and his blindness is due to maculopathy. He is currently having the following recommended devices: OD: -4.25 -3.50 X 010, OS: -4.25 -4.00 X 160, illuminated handheld magnifier 6.5 X / 22D PWR MAG SPT and monocular telescope PD 36, 38 OS. CCTV SRX OD: -1.75 -3.50 X 010 OS: -1.75 -4.00 X 160 5D LUXO LAMP with +10D Loupe, Floor Stand, and Casters.

LESSON OBJECTIVE: Mr. Fritz will be introduced to stovetop safety, cleanup prevention, cleanup, flipping, spreading and checking doneness techniques.

All materials and equipment needed for the training were available at the client's house

STEPS TAUGHT / STEPS PROVIDED: I provided an orientation to the stove top controls and discussed selecting a burner and keeping the handle of the pan away from the edge of the countertop. Safety zone technique, Non-visual monitoring techniques were discussed using smell and hearing to listen to progression of cooked food. Adaptive spreading techniques were also shown including using a spoon for spreading soft margarine from the center out to the edges. A double-sided spatula was used for added control while flipping. I advised the client that I will order and issue him the double spatula at my next visit.

SUCCESS OF INSTRUCTION: Mr. Fritz was able to prepare a grilled cheese sandwich on the stovetop using the techniques shown. He reported difficulty with using twist ties on bread bags. Alternatives techniques were discussed for sealing bread. He also had some difficulty operating heating controls. The addition of high visibility labels at home would help him identify controls easier.

BARRIERS (IF ANY): Reduced hand dexterity

CLEARANCE/SAFETY ISSUES (IF ANY): Mr. Fritz has the potential of being burned while handling hot pans and foods.

NEXT CLASS OBJECTIVE: Adaptive oven safety techniques including opening and closing oven door, pulling out oven rack, centering pan onto rack, and removing item from oven. Provide an overview of oven controls and adaptive timing

4. **Background:** Jonathan is 46-year-old Caucasian American male, diagnosed with diabetic retinopathy, glaucoma, Unspecified Hearing Loss, Dementia, 20/400 OD, and 20/800 OS. His current reading Prescription: Plano (pl.) – 1:00 X 45 OD and Pl. -1.50 X 135 and tint: amber 90% transmission. He was referred to our Low Vision and Blind Facility (PCVI=Prince Center for Visually Impaired) for an introduction to the slate and stylus in order to prepare for a braille lesson.

Lesson objective: Introduction to slate and stylus

Materials needed: Slate and Stylus (provided by PCVI), index card, eraser and lighting

Instruction provided: Jonathan was introduced to slate and stylus. He was directed to punch out full cells for practice, and then wrote out the braille alphabet, then wrote words using the letters A-h.

Success of instruction: Jonathan was able to punch out full cells for practice and wrote out the braille alphabet with verbal assistance. He was able to write words using the letters A-h independently. He checked the words he wrote for accuracy. Jonathan followed instruction well and understands the concept of the slate and stylus.

Clearance/safety issuer if any: None

Next class objective: Review Slate and Stylus

5. **Background:** Jonathan is 46-year-old Caucasian American male, diagnosed with diabetic retinopathy, glaucoma, Unspecified Hearing Loss, Dementia, 20/400 OD, and 20/800 OS. His current reading Prescription: Plano (pl.) – 1:00 X 45 OD and Pl. -1.50 X 135 and tint: amber 90% transmission.

Goal: Learn braille reading techniques.

Lesson objective: To have the veteran tactually read the Braille letters J and I.

Steps taught/instruction provided: Jonathan continued reading various letters, words and phrases relating to the letters J and I. He was reminded to relax his hand and to choose one finger to read the letters instead of switching between his thumb, index and middle fingers.

Success of instruction: Jonathan was able to successfully read the words and one phrase with little difficulty.

Barriers if any: none

Clearance/safety issue: none

Next class objective: Continue with Braille reading techniques.

6. **Background:** Mrs. FR is 91, diagnosed with AMD OD and Leukocoria OS. She was born with this impairment. Her visual acuity was 20/400 OD and 20/800 OS. New York State Commission for the blind referred her to our organization for Vocational Rehabilitation services. I was mandated to continue one of her lesson training on the Reizen Talking Calculator originally scheduled by a CVRT who was off that day.

Review of Talking Calculator

Instruction provided: Mrs. FR continued to learn Talking calculator. She reviewed some of the large print addition, subtraction, multiplication, division problems using the calculator. She was also introduced to the percentage key and completed some of the percentage problems.

Success of Instruction: Mrs. FR became more familiar with the buttons on the calculator. She has been issued his talking calculator and large print math problems to complete over the weekend.

Barriers: none

7. **Background:** Mr. JC is 94-year-old African American male, diagnosed with AMD OU. With eccentric viewing at 4:00 and short-term memory loss. This training was done at Mr. JC's home.

LESSON OBJECTIVE: Introduction to the talking books library services and digital talking book machine.

STEPS TAUGHT / STEPS PROVIDED: I introduced him the talking books services and digital talking books machine.

SUCCESS OF INSTRUCTION: Mr. JC was able to successfully follow along with the instruction material presented. He was able to visually locate the power, play, fast-forward, rewind, sleep, tone, and speed buttons. He was also able to independently insert a new talking book cartridge into the player and listen to the book.

BARRIERS (IF ANY): none

CLEARANCE/SAFETY ISSUES (IF ANY): none

NEXT CLASS OBJECTIVE: Review Olympus digital voice recorder

8. **Background:** Mr. JC is 94-year-old African American male, diagnosed with AMD OU. With eccentric viewing at 4:00 and short-term memory loss. This training was done at Mr. JC's home.

Lesson Objective: Review Olympus digital voice recorder

Instruction provided: Reviewed with him the Olympus Digital recorder by recording and erasing messages. Mr. JC reviewed use of the record, play, stop and erase, rewind, fast-forward and folders buttons on the device.

Success of Instruction: JC was able to complete recording, playing messages. He was able to record and erase messages in each of his folders. An Olympus Digital Recorder will be ordered for him. Also reviewed setting of his time and alarm on his 4 button Atomic talking watch.

Barriers: None

Next class objective: Review clocks.

9. **Background:** Mr. CB is 88-year-old, diagnosed with diabetic retinopathy and glaucoma. He also has a hearing impairment in his right ear. His visual acuity was 20/400 OD and 20/800 OS. Here again, I was mandated to work with Mr. CB with his new Norelco electric shaver.

Lucien G Prince, MD, MBA,MS-CVRT, CLVT

Lesson objective: Introduce Norelco electric shaver. Review basic operation and maintenance of the electric razor.

Instruction provided: I reviewed the Norelco shaver with him and covered shaving with an electric razor, charging and cleaning of the shaver.

Success of Instruction: Mr. CB understood how to use and clean the shaver. I also issued him his low vision black face watch and headphones.

Barriers: none

References

1. Sterns GK, Hyvarinen L. Adressing Pediatric Issues. In: Fletcher DC. *Low Vision Rehabilitation: Caring for the Whole Person.* American Academy of Ophthalmology. 1999. 107-119.
2. Faye EE. Clinical Low Vision. 2a. Ed. Boston/Toronto: Little, Brown, and Company. 1984.
3. Watson GR. Using Low Vision Effectively. In: Fletcher DC. *Low Vision Rehabilitation: Caring for the Whole Person.* American Academy of Ophthalmology. 1999. 61-87.
4. Hyvarinen L, Jacob N. What and How Does this Child See? Assessment of Visual Functioning for Development and Learning. Helsinki, Finland: Vistest Ltd. 2011. 174.
5. Colenbrander A, Liegner JT, Fletcher DC. Enhancing Impaired Vision. In: Fletcher DC. *Low Vision Rehabilitation: Caring for the Whole Person.* American Academy of Ophthalmology. 1999. 49-59.
6. Brilliant R. (1999). Essential of Low Vision Practice. Butterworth-Heineman, MA
7. Course Materials-Salus University-Kerry Lueders 2014
8. *Ponchillia P. & Ponchillia S. (1996). Foundations of Rehabilitation Teaching with Persons who are Blind or Visually impaired. AFB. PRESS. New York, NY.*
9. Orr, L. (1992) Vision and Aging. Crossroads for Services Delivery. AFP Press New York NY
10. Lachelle Smith (2015) Course materials Salus University
11. *Ponchillia P. (1996) Foundations of Rehabilitations teaching AFB Press New York NY*
12. *Orr, a & Rogers P. (2003) Solutions for Success – AFB Press New York NY*
13. *Presley I & D'Andrea F. (2008) Assistive Technology for Students who are blind or visually impaired – AFB Press New York, NY*
14. *Loumiet, R. & Levack, N. (1993). Independent Living. 2nd ed. Texas School for the Blind and Visually Impaired Austin, TX*
    http://www.aoa.org/patients-and-public/caring-for-your-vision/comprehensive-eye-and-vision-examination/limitations-of-vision-screening-programs?sso=y
    http://www.lighthouse.org/for-professionals/practice-management/structured-low-vision-exam
    http://www.massoptom.org/images/customer-files/lowvisionexamnotes.pdf
    http://www.lowvision.org/what_occurs_in_a_low_vision_exam.htm
    http://www.ski.org/Colenbrander/Images/Low_Vision_Exam.pdf
    www.bucksblind.org/my_files/**low vision exams**.pps
    https://www.youtube.com/watch?v=QQw20Rc9J6Q
    http://www.petroueyecare.com/eye-care-services/low-vision-exam/
    http://www.aoa.org/patients-and-public/caring-for-your-vision/low-vision/low-vision-exam?sso=y

http://www.meade.com/support/power.html
http://www.visionaware.org/info/your-eye-condition/eye-health/low-vision/low-vision-examination/1235
http://www.lighthouse.org/about-low-vision-blindness/braving-low-vision-exam/
http://www.ninds.nih.gov/disorders/autism/detail_autism.htm#259233082
http://www.emstac.org/registered/topics/autism/case.htm
http://www.emstac.org/registered/topics/autism/case.htm
http://en.wikipedia.org/wiki/Lovaas_model
http://www.autismspeaks.org/family-services/resource-library/assistive-technology

Index

Printed in the United States
By Bookmasters